Also by Dr. Phil McGraw

Life Code

Real Life

Love Smart

Family First

Family First Workbook

The Ultimate Weight Solution

The Ultimate Weight Solution Cookbook

The Ultimate Weight Solution Food Guide

Self Matters

Self Matters Companion

Relationship Rescue

Relationship Rescue Workbook

Life Strategies

Life Strategies Workbook

THE
20/20
DIET

Turn Your Weight Loss Vision into Reality

20 Key Foods to Help You
Succeed Where Other Diets Fail

Dr. Phil McGraw

Published in Los Angeles, California, by Bird Street Books, Inc.

ISBN: Print   978-1-939457-31-8
      EPub   978-1-939457-30-1
      Mobi   978-1-939457-29-5
      PDF   978-1-939457-28-8

Cover Design: Longerday.com
Interior Design: Stuart Smith
Interior Production: Dovetail Publishing Services

I dedicate this book to all the people who have had a lifetime ticket on the weight loss rollercoaster but never give up trying to get in shape and return to health. My sincere wish is that you will use this plan to finally free yourself from your weight burden and start living the life you truly deserve.

Note to Readers

The anecdotes in this book are used to illustrate common issues and problems that I have encountered and do not necessarily portray specific people or situations. No real names have been used.

As with all books, this one contains opinions and ideas of the author. It is intended to provide helpful and informative material on the subjects addressed in the publication. It is sold with the understanding that the author and publisher are not engaged in rendering medical, health, psychological, or any other kind of personal professional services or therapy in the book. The reader should consult his or her medical, health, psychological, or other competent professional before adopting any of the concepts in this book or drawing inferences from it. The content of this book, by its very nature, is general, whereas each reader's situation is unique. Therefore, as with all books of this nature, the purpose is to provide general information rather than address individual situations, which books by their very nature cannot do.

The author and publisher specifically disclaim all responsibility for any liability, loss, or risk, personal or otherwise, which is incurred as a consequence, directly or indirectly, of the use and application of any of the contents of this book.

ACKNOWLEDGMENTS

First, I want to thank my beautiful wife, Robin. For 40 years I have witnessed you living every day with such passion for health and well-being. Leading by example, you inspire not only me, but also anyone in your pathway, to live healthfully and be better people.

I thank our sons, Jay and Jordan. You give your parents powerful reasons to take care of ourselves, and inspire us by your own pursuit of excellence.

Thanks to Cynthia Sass, M.P.H, R.D, whose nutritional expertise is evident in all of the meals and menus in this book. Her tireless work creating just the right balance of nutrients was invaluable. And I know readers will appreciate her formal culinary training because her detailed attention to taste makes the meals within these pages truly come to life on their plates.

Thanks to Maggie Greenwood-Robinson, Ph.D., for once again lending your nutrition, exercise, and superb research skills to this project. You always raise the bar on content and I appreciate your contributions to this book.

I acknowledge my friend and colleague G. Frank Lawlis, Ph.D., A.B.P.P., a fellow of the American Psychological Association and chairman of the advisory board for the *Dr. Phil* show. Thanks for all the wisdom you have imparted and for being there for me both personally and professionally for nearly 40 years including your counsel in the science of health management.

Carla Pennington, thank you for being at the helm of the *Dr. Phil* show team. I appreciate your daily commitment to excellence as we work with so many deserving individuals and families. Thank you, in specific, for your input on this book and creating so many teachable moments about health on the show.

And I extend a very special thanks to my good friend and colleague, Joey Carson, as well as the entire team at Bird Street Books, especially Lisa Clark for her patience and tireless efforts on this project over the last two years. Lisa, you were the absolute key to making this book a reality. You were a relentless researcher, editor, planner, organizer, and "cleaner upper." Thank you for your role in creating a responsible data-based book.

To Oprah Winfrey, my dear friend, thank you for creating the opportunity and platform for Dr. Phil. My family and I will always be grateful for you.

CONTENTS

INTRODUCTION

You create the results in life that you believe you deserve.
—Dr. Phil McGraw

I'm betting if you honored me by acquiring this book, you already know enough about me to realize that I am going to tell you the unvarnished truth, at least as I see it, whether it is what you *want* to hear or not. If that's your thinking, then you're right. The way I see it is if you spend your time and money with me, then I owe you nothing less than the truth you *need* to hear in order to get what you want.

There is an old saying: "BS the fans, *not* the players!" I want to be on your team here. I want you to be a player—a smart, savvy player—and I want to play this "weight game" with you. I want to help you get *real results*. So here we go! Let's do this right, lose the weight consistently and in a healthy manner, and learn diet strategies to last a lifetime.

When it comes to your weight and health, I see that you have three choices:

1. You can choose to be in denial about your weight problem.
2. You can choose to fall for another "eat what you want and still get thin" lie.
3. You can choose to lose weight in a healthy manner with diet strategies that you can use for the rest of your life.

If you chose the last option, I wrote this book for you. I want to help you transform your body, your *body image*, your lifestyle, your priorities, and your self-worth, all in one fell swoop. To neglect *any* part of that list is to set you up for failure.

But you have to be honest with yourself *right now*, right from the beginning. You may just be going through the motions here, *acting* like you want to and will lose weight, but in truth, in that most honest part of your psyche, you're thinking, "I will never really lose weight. I am a failure at this, but if I don't at least act like I am trying, then I will feel like a complete pig loser!" Or you might be thinking, "Oh, I'm just too far gone. Too late, Dr. Phil! I'm a lost cause!"

My own sister Deana told me last year that she was so fat that it took two dogs to bark at her! She said when it was hot outside, people were gathering on her shady side. As usual, she was masking her pain with jokes. Funny, but not slimming. She is even bigger today than she was last year. So, maybe three dogs now? (Ouch! She will make me pay for that!)

My whole family has always struggled with weight. This time last year, I had two nephews who each weighed close to 500 pounds. One of them told me, "Uncle Phil, I'm dying a slow death here. I am a recluse. I have no life. I'm not living; I'm merely existing. I am a grown man, yet I have no social life, I haven't been on a date in years, and I'm ashamed of myself every time I look in the mirror. I hide in shame and I am so lonely and discouraged that my days feel a week long. I go out late at night to get fast food and come back and eat it alone. It's pathetic. I have to make my last stand right now or I know I will be dead in months. I can barely breathe. I am afraid, I am *really* afraid. I am to the point where I would rather be dead than live this way. I am ready to change this, really ready. Please help me and I promise I will not disappoint you or myself."

I believed him, he *was* ready, and I did help. Because he needed constant medical supervision while working to shed the extra pounds (as any extreme weight loss should be done under the supervision of a doctor), I sent him to a facility where he could focus full-time on reclaiming his health. In the last year, he has lost over 200 pounds! His health has improved greatly; he has gotten off all his medications for diabetes, hypertension, and so on. He has gone from not being able to walk from one room to the next without great difficulty to walking and jogging five miles a day out in the fresh air. He has become an avid golfer and is dating a lovely young woman he met while on his quest.

His brother, on the other hand, did nothing different than what got him to almost 500 pounds and guess what happened to him? Wait for it . . . he got bigger. But, and this is a big but (no pun intended), inspired by his younger brother, he tells me *he* is ready now, and I know he means it. For the first time, he really means it. His time has come.

How about you? Are you ready? Has *your* time come? Is this the moment that you will look back on and say, "I can tell you exactly the moment I decided enough was enough. The exact moment I decided I was not going to take this from myself anymore. The exact moment I claimed my right to become master of my body and my mind and create the results I so desperately wanted, yet cheated myself out of."

I believe we all come to critical junctures in life, when we are at a precipice where all things wrong can be made right. Let this be your moment in time. The past is over, the future hasn't happened yet, the only time is right now. This can be your threshold moment of change. The next year of your life is going to go by whether you're doing something about your weight or not. Now, think about what I just said: the next year is going to go by. You cannot stop the march of time. Choose denial and you will just get bigger and bigger. Ply yourself with too-good-to-be-true schemes and you will just get bigger and bigger.

Don't let days turn into weeks, weeks turn into months, and months turn into years while you sit around not doing something that you are fully and totally capable of doing. You can do this! I promise you that you can, even if you have doubts. Since the next year of your life is going to go by whether you are doing something about your weight or not, now is the time to get started.

I'm not going to insult your intelligence by blowing smoke at you and telling you it will be automatic or even what you might call easy. If I did, you would know better in your heart of hearts, even if you chose to believe me. So instead of conning you or helping you con yourself, I want you to know right up front that, just as my nephew did, you're going to have to change several aspects of your life. This does not mean that you will feel like you are in prison or being punished with hunger and deprivation, but there will be big changes. When you're ready, and I mean really ready, to make the necessary changes, you'll be surprised how doable it all is.

First, you're going to have to *stop using food for anything other than nutrition*. You cannot continue to use food to celebrate, or as a companion, or for entertainment, or comfort. You cannot medicate yourself, your mood, or pain with food.

It is a simple but profound resolve: let's agree to deal with psychological problems psychologically, medical problems medically, and social problems socially. Come on, let's be real. If some schmuck broke your heart because you caught him sexting with some Silicone Sally from work, you know you can't fix it by bonding with Ben and Jerry! (By the way, you probably already knew he was a schmuck.)

My point is, you aren't overweight because you use food; you are overweight, at least in part, because you *misuse* food. Cheese puffs won't fix your problems. I wish they could; I would go into the cheese puffs business and become a billionaire! You need to eat to live, not live to eat. You need to feed your body, not your fat. Even dumb animals do it! Think about it: Have you ever, *ever* seen a *fat* coyote? How about a fat mountain lion? No, you have not! They are hunters, good hunters, and they eat what they *need* and go do whatever it is coyotes and mountain lions do. Mountain lions don't go and eat an extra deer because the cat in the next tree has a prettier coat of fur or was hanging out with *her* tomcat.

Next resolve: you've got to *stop being a sucker*! People can tell you, "Eat everything you want and lose weight!" Come on, really?! Or they'll tell you about the new fad "kumquat soup diet" or "cabbage and cardboard diet." If you believe all of that, then you are a "Double D": dumb and desperate. That is the wrong kind of Double D. You know better. You know the truth when you hear it, right? The truth is, you have to be willing to make some changes and, yes, you have to be willing to make some sacrifices. Unless and until you stop using food for anything other than nutrition and stop believing infomercial hype, you're not going to lose weight and create habits that can help keep it off. Sorry! It doesn't matter if you do this diet or 10 others: if you don't get real with yourself, you simply will not have the results you deserve.

Also critical to this mission is honing in on the mistakes and missteps of your past. As the old saying goes, hindsight is 20/20. We all see things more clearly the morning after. There's a reason Monday morning quarterbacks have all the answers—they've got the benefit of having already seen the whole game! That's exactly what you and I need to do, because the mistakes you've made over the years hold the clues to getting it right this time. Let's also look beyond your own setbacks at some of the common reasons other people fail on diets. I am confident that you will see yourself reflected somewhere in that list, and you will finally understand why you haven't been able to succeed at losing weight despite your numerous attempts.

Then I want you to take it a step further and have *foresight* that is 20/20. It may be hard for you to imagine how your life will change, because it's a goal you've only ever dreamed of in the abstract. But you must have a clear vision of what it will look, smell, taste, and feel like when you proudly cross the finish line. Or, more accurately, the starting line, because it's the beginning of an entirely new landscape for you when you look and feel the way you deserve.

Let's get specific. How will it feel when you aren't fighting your clothes all day because they actually fit? And what emotions will you experience when you see your new body reflected in the mirror? How will your relationship with your family change when you're able to keep up with the kids at the park or simply get your chores done without becoming out of breath? Let's get right down to how every detail of your day-to-day life will change and then follow that vision all the way to reality by using the tools I'm giving you.

I'm bringing this book out more than 10 years after my first book on this same topic, *The Ultimate Weight Solution*. In that one, I talked about the "seven keys of weight loss freedom." I've woven all of them into the fabric of this diet, and (and this is an important "and") I have gone well beyond *The Ultimate Weight Solution* because emerging research and new theories provide new information about how your body processes and reacts to food. As a result, this book includes some new information and theories from bariatric research (i.e., the study of obesity) that are important to the science of weight management.

You will be shocked at some of the revelations, especially those involving genetics and biochemistry, because they may help explain why, despite your best efforts, your body has been unwilling to shed excess fat deposits. New research and theories have also yielded helpful information about certain common foods and specific exercise patterns that I believe may be able to help you in your efforts to lose weight. I'm excited about these new tools, and I think you will be too.

My goal is to bring you the newest information along with time-proven keys for success. Paramount among those keys is "healing feelings." That's what I mean when I say you cannot use food for anything other than nutrition. You've got to resolve your emotional needs rather than react to them by eating. I repeat: you can't deal with a psychological, social, financial, romantic, or any other kind of problem with food.

Another key is "right thinking." If you don't get your mind and behavior right, you will never get your body right—you will never lose the weight and adopt the lifelong behaviors needed to keep it off. I've already started adjusting your thinking—by opening your eyes to the idea that every pie-in-the-sky diet or weight loss product on the market isn't the magical cure for your weight problem. I intend to manipulate your thinking by showing you the truth about those empty promises, those diet mirages that you keep chasing.

Have you ever seen an actual mirage? Plenty of times driving down Texas roads on days so hot that even the trees are looking for shade, I've seen what looks like a sparkling puddle of water on the asphalt a little ways ahead of my car. But as I get closer to it, it vanishes. It's called a highway mirage, and it's an optical phenomenon caused by a combination of the hot air just above the road and a refraction of the sun's rays that create a mirror effect. Our brains fill in the blanks and tell us that there's a puddle of water a hundred yards down the road. It's a false image, an illusion.

But it's so convincing, right? I mean, this "water" is reflecting oncoming traffic. It seems to have movement. It has all the qualities of a perfectly good puddle, but in actuality, the ground is dry as can be. How could your mind play a trick on you like that?

When you think about it, certain elements of the weight loss industry aren't so different from a mirage. Those advertisements you see for pills, powders, systems, products, and programs that promise weight loss without diet, exercise, or lifestyle changes are all very convincing.

I'll bet right off the top of your head, you can think of at least 10 different "miracle" products that claim to shrink waistlines, sculpt muscles, or melt fat, many of which you've tried. They're presented with just enough pseudoscience to help your brain make the leap, fill in the blanks, and buy into the illusion. It all sounds so technical, logical, and real. So you press the "buy" button with the very best of intentions, you try them out, and maybe you lose a few pounds, maybe you don't. (If you did lose some weight, it was probably a placebo effect just from being focused on it for a while.) Either way, before you know what happened, you're right back where you started, or worse off with some extra poundage hanging out around your waist or hips because you had a false sense of security and ate anything that was dead or seriously slowed down. Smoke, mirrors, and very clever (not to mention expensive) marketing suckered you in. Again.

You're not alone—far from it. Americans spend $61 billion each year on weight loss products. This is a $61 billion-a-year industry with quite a few "miracle" products that don't work! How is that possible? If you had roller skates that wouldn't skate, surfboards that wouldn't surf, and cars that wouldn't drive, you would not continue to buy those products. You'd be outraged! But diets that don't work? No problem! Millions of people line up to spend billions of dollars because they're desperate for the magic bullet easy fix.

Maybe you're persuaded by one of those celebrities you see showing off his or her new, svelte look while touting diet programs and weight loss products on TV commercials. Would you like to take a stab at guessing how much they're *paid* to lose that weight? The average range is probably between $500,000 and a cool $3 million. I'll bet if someone offered you a couple million bucks to lose weight, you'd pretty much eat sawdust and chain yourself to the treadmill to earn that paycheck.

Until that offer comes your way, I want you to stop deluding yourself. Those "miracle" weight loss products and programs you've been using aren't for weight loss; they're gimmicks. You've been obsessing about your weight and compulsively dieting, maybe for years. Obsession is thought, compulsion is behavior, and we have a generation of obsessive-compulsive dieters. Why don't we stop the insanity? You need to be mature enough to recognize that weight goes on a lot

Listen to Your Gut

The Federal Trade Commission (FTC), a government agency whose motto is "Protecting America's Consumers," urges the media to have their radar up for too-good-to-be-true weight loss scams. Before featuring a weight loss product on the air, the FTC has asked that media outlets consider seven "gut check claims," which are statements commonly made in bogus weight loss product ads. Unfortunately, not everyone complies, and you'll still see commercials, infomercials, and TV segments on many products making these kinds of outrageous statements.

I think these seven gut check claims are valid, and I want you to be armed with them too. Don't be a sucker for ridiculous products designed to do nothing but cost you money, and sometimes even your health. Beware of weight loss products that claim to:

1. cause weight loss of two pounds or more a week for a month or more without dieting or exercise;
2. cause substantial weight loss no matter what or how much the consumer eats;
3. cause permanent weight loss even after the consumer stops using the product;
4. block the absorption of fat or calories to enable consumers to lose substantial weight;
5. safely enable consumers to lose more than three pounds per week for more than four weeks;
6. cause substantial weight loss for all users; or
7. cause substantial weight loss by wearing a product on the body or rubbing it into the skin.

If you hear someone make any of these claims for a weight loss product, supplement, drug, patch, cream, wrap, and so on, you are being ripped off. There is no magic bullet for weight loss, no overnight cure. If it doesn't involve a healthy, balanced diet and a reasonable exercise regimen, it will not lead to safe weight loss. End of story!

easier than it comes off, and if you find a diet that works, then you will lose weight while you're on it. Now ask yourself if you're really going to spend the rest of your life on one of those ridiculous diets. The honest answer is, no, you won't. So, that means you might lose weight while you're on it, but you'll probably gain it back when you're off it because you haven't made any real lifestyle changes.

My goal is to get you to stop chasing diet mirages and finally get yourself on the right path, with the habits you should follow for life to achieve permanent weight loss. Bottom line: if it sounds too good to be true, it is. Yes, there's a lot of noise out there; there's literally a new "diet of the week" every week! But now is the time to quit being a sheep and a sucker.

Now, I'm not saying that every diet and exercise plan on the market is some kind of con. There are plenty of viable (and healthy) weight loss systems out there. But maybe you've faced failure even with the *healthy* ones. Why? That's what I wanted to know when I began researching this book, because knowing why something *doesn't* work is equally as important as knowing why it does. You remember the story about Thomas Edison creating the light bulb? It took him a thousand or more tries, but as he famously said, "I have not failed. I've just found 10,000 ways that won't work." Then he used that information to find out what *did* work. Bingo, let there be light. If ever there was a man who learned from his 20/20 hindsight, it was him! And you're about to embark on a similar path as you learn from your own past, failures and all.

If you're fighting a weight problem and you bought this book, you've probably been overweight for a long time and you've probably tried to lose it more times than you can remember. I conducted a national survey of my viewers, social media followers, and others that garnered thousands of responses, and now we've all got the opportunity to learn from each other's histories. I found out that 40.3 percent of you have lost weight on diets and gained 100% of it back within 90 days to one year. I really wanted to know—why do people fail on diets so much of the time? So we asked people what got in their way. When you watch those commercials on TV, they don't tell you why you're going to fail; they just tell you how great everything's going to be. But you deserve the truth, so I set out to find it.

Sure enough, I found seven reasons why people failed to lose weight that I thought I could help you with in this diet. Here they are:

1. **Hunger:** You get tired of feeling hungry all the time. So you rebel.

2. **Cravings:** You consistently crave certain tastes like salty, sweet, or tart. So you rebel.

3. **Feelings of restriction:** You feel like you can't eat out, go anywhere, or do anything because you're on a diet. Plus, you're so panicked about what you can and can't eat and when you should or shouldn't eat it that your focus on food becomes all-consuming. So you rebel.

4. **Impracticality and expense:** Between your job, the kids, stress, and life—you feel like you just can't get it all done *and* stick to a diet, especially one that's too complicated, expensive, and requires you to count calories or nutritional values. So you rebel.

5. **Boredom:** You get sick of eating the same foods day in and day out. So you rebel.

6. **Temptations:** Because your environment isn't fail-safe, you are overwhelmed by your desire for the tempting food all around you. So you rebel.

7. **Inconsistent results and plateaus:** You get discouraged because the weight loss is not consistent. Or you lose weight for a while but then your progress comes to a screeching halt. So you rebel.

Now, that's a lot of rebellion! I knew if you and I were going to get along, then I had to solve these seven problems for you. I had to design a plan that would not be sabotaged by these seven flaws that have caused many others to fail to reach their weight loss goals. And that's exactly what this diet is designed to do. I knew that if you were going to succeed, this diet had to find solutions to these seven "rebellion triggers" so that your experience would include:

- **Decreased hunger**
- **Decreased cravings**

- **No sense of restriction**
- **A diet you can live with**
- **No boredom**
- **A no-fail environment**
- **Consistent weight loss and a system to help you address plateaus**

How is all that possible? As I said, since *The Ultimate Weight Solution* came out over 10 years ago, new research and theories have emerged that allow me to do an even more effective job of helping you solve these seven problems. This is really exciting: research continues to provide us with important new theories about how certain foods and activities affect our bodies and brains. In this book, I've harnessed this information and provided you with practical tips that I think you can easily incorporate into your lifestyle to help you with your weight loss journey today and for the rest of your life.

For starters, you will be eating 20 key foods called the 20/20 Foods, which developing research suggests may:

☑ *Help increase your body's thermogenesis.*

☑ *Help you feel fuller* when you eat them so that you feel satisfied and you're not leaving the table hungry. If you are so hungry your stomach is barbequing your ribs, guess what? You *will rebel!* If you don't feel that way, *you won't.*

☑ *Have a "time-release" effect*, which means they can help you feel full for longer *after* eating them, so you're not starving to death and craving every doughnut you see.

And that's just the beginning. On top of this, you'll be doing a type of exercise that recent research and theories suggest is fast, efficient, and can help keep you on track to meet your weight loss goals. We'll talk more about the nuts and bolts of this plan and the research behind all of it a little later.

So, my job in this book is to address these seven problems, and your job is to get real about why you're overeating and to start believing that you deserve to lose weight and be healthy. Because if you *believe*, and I mean really believe, that you deserve better, you will *create* better for yourself. If you don't believe you deserve better, then you won't get better. That's why I started this introduction with this statement: *you create the results in life that you believe you deserve.*

What I want to do in this book is tell you the truth. You've read the rest, now here's the best. You can go try all those other products and programs that promise weight loss without diet and exercise all you want and feel really good in the moment, but six months from now, you're likely going to weigh the same as you do right now—or more—and you know it. Or you can let me tell you what you should do cognitively, behaviorally, environmentally, socially, and nutritionally, and you can adopt these habits for a lifetime of healthy weight. You can choose to see your goal with 20/20 accuracy, and when you can see a goal that clearly, you can achieve it.

We're in this together, so let's get going.

1

WHAT MAKES THIS DIET DIFFERENT

Great things are not done by impulse,
but by a series of small things brought together.
—Vincent Van Gogh

There are no two ways about it: managing weight is frustrating. Unless you are one of those "gene pool lottery winners" who got the metabolism and body type of a greyhound on speed, then you (and I, by the way) have to contend with the tendency to gain weight. I can practically just walk by French fries or smell a chocolate cake and gain 10 pounds! And that's not totally in jest, because I am genetically predisposed to be overweight and the experts tell me that if I even smell certain foods, my brain reacts in a way that impacts the efficiency with which my body processes food. I am a classic "weight loss resistant" patient, and you may be too. (Even if you are among the small percentage of people who fit the bill, it is NOT an excuse to be overweight; it just means you have a somewhat different set of challenges. You can expect much, much more on that later.) But either way, medically weight loss resistant or not, I'm betting you feel like you've been on a chaotic, never-ending merry-go-round of diets and you just can't get your body to cooperate. Am I right?

If you just got stupid one day and hopped in an airplane cockpit, somehow got the plane to take off, instantly crashed, hopped back in (BIG stupid), took off, and instantly crashed again, then continued to do it over and over—at some point limping away from your wreck of an airplane with a broken propeller under one arm and a tree branch under the other, wouldn't you eventually say to yourself,

"Hey, dummy, you might want to take the time and *learn to fly* before you do this again!" You may be "hopping in" but you are damn sure "limping away"! The pattern is clear: all you know how to do is crash.

Are you doing the same thing in your attempts at losing weight—hopping into diet after diet and crashing? Maybe that's really why they call them "crash diets"! Ha! Well, I want you to stop being a crasher and start being a winner. If you figure out *why* you're crashing and use that 20/20 hindsight to your advantage, chances are pretty good you will stop doing whatever it is that isn't working, even if *not* crashing is harder to do. I have often said that the difference between winners and losers is that winners do things losers just don't want to do. It's hard, no question. And it takes a big commitment. It is time to choose winning.

We already know that you've got to stop chasing after get-thin-quick diet mirages, but now let's take a close look at precisely why they fail you. These are the Top Seven "Ugly Truths" about Dieting derived from the survey we discussed in the introduction, where people just like you told us exactly why they failed again and again. After each ugly truth, I will show you exactly how I am going to help you overcome it once and for all with habits to last a lifetime.

The Top Seven "Ugly Truths" about Dieting

Hunger

Fact: Hungry people eat. You leave the table feeling unsatisfied and by the time evening rolls around, you're ready to eat the paint off the walls. So what happens? You binge. Hungry people are eventually going to eat, and eat with a vengeance! We are programmed to eat so we can survive as a species, for Pete's sake. Come on, a diet that starves you, one that leaves you hungry all or even most of the time, is just a crap diet. It is seriously flawed because it goes against human nature. And then you feel guilty for behaving precisely the way nature has programmed you. That guilt (for behaving normally) crowds out motivation and self-confidence and damages your personal truth, and that's when the slide begins. **Result: Failure.**

With this plan, I've got to get you to where you don't feel imprisoned by constant, gnawing hunger. This is not rocket science—when you get naturally hungry, you need to have something to eat. Apparently nobody has really bothered to think about the fact that you simply cannot go hungry on a diet! The first thing you will learn is how to distinguish between actual, physical hunger (defined as your body's true need for nutrition) and "mind hunger," which is really just a response to a trigger, emotional or otherwise. This is fundamental: you must tune in to your body and its needs and, as I have said, respond to emotional needs emotionally and physical needs physically. Once you've identified which needs are which and learned to respond accordingly, you've fought 90 percent of the battle. I will give you my Hunger and Fullness Scale, which is an essential tool to help you recognize whether your body really needs food or if you're just experiencing fake hunger in reaction to a trigger or out of habit. If it's the latter, I'll also show you how to keep from giving in and sabotaging yourself.

As for nutrition, it's likely you will need to reduce your current portions in order to lose weight. But reducing your portions from the gargantuan sizes you (and the rest of America, by the way) might be eating now to a proper, healthy, weight-loss–inducing size does not mean you have to be hungry. Why? Because it's not just about eating less; it's about eating more of the *right* foods. That's why the dietitians that helped design this plan have looked at the latest theories and emerging research to find foods for this program that can help you feel fuller at mealtime and sustain that feeling after you've eaten. When you're feeling true, physical hunger, rest assured, you will have plenty to eat on this plan. **Result: Success.**

Cravings

If you were a drug addict and you quit cold turkey, you'd experience withdrawals. As you are starting this diet, you are very likely addicted to other types of "drugs": sugar, simple carbohydrates, salt, or fat. But you weren't born craving a Twinkie or a bag of greasy chips. You *learned* that palate. Here's the bright side: I believe anything you can learn, you can *un*learn.

Certain diets simply don't address that! They just throw you in the deep end and don't teach you how to swim. They expect you to quit all your food addictions cold turkey and give you no plan or hope for dealing with the cravings you will go through. Then it's only a matter of time until you give in, and guess what? Rebellion. Before you know it, you're making your third trip to the 24-hour convenience store to get some "convenient" food (translation: you can eat it like a wood chipper grinding up balsa wood and give yourself a gut bomb you couldn't process in a week). Or maybe you find yourself waking up in the middle of the night and walking, zombie-like, into the kitchen for a colossal pig-out session. You're like those gremlins in that movie who went nuts when they ate after midnight! Just like a drug addict, you feel defenseless against your ever-increasing need for a fix. **Result: Failure.**

They don't tell you in other diets that you're most likely going to have some withdrawals at first, but if you just bear down for a few days, they should diminish. Whether your addictions are psychological or physiological, they should diminish. But by not explaining this to you, they leave you feeling hopeless, like there's no end in sight. There was a study done years ago in which researchers told one group of subjects they were going to introduce a painful stimulus until they were through with the test, and then they'd get $10 for their trouble. They told another group the same thing, *except* that there was a panic button they could hit at any time so if the pain became too much, they could stop it. Well, the group who knew they were in control of when it would stop could take four or five times more pain than the other group who were just promised a reward in the end. The same is true with your cravings.

In this plan, I'm going to help you get over your cravings by giving you specific foods to help ease them, and I'm going to give you specific foods to help ease your cravings for junk food. You have learned to like those unhealthy foods, but you *can* change your palate. Once that happens, you'll look back and think, "OMG, I can't believe I was eating that!" That morning pastry you used to think was terrific will taste like you just bit into a hunk of lard that's so sweet it's sickening. I will try to help you get to that point through powerful insight *and* encouraging you to eat certain foods that are at least categorically related to your craving so that you can satisfy that need in the interim. **Result: Success.**

Feelings of restriction

Certain diets have lists (long ones!) of "taboo" foods—ones that you absolutely, categorically, cannot eat no matter what. Simply stated, that tactic leads to rebellion. Here's how it usually plays out: You feel restricted, like you're stuck on this unbearable diet forever and you'll never be allowed to eat a piece of bread or a steak ever again in your life. Then you feel sorry for yourself, like you're being punished, like you can't go out with friends, enjoy the holidays, or go on a vacation. It's as though all the fun has been removed from your life—like you're missing out on everything because you're "on a diet." And that's when the first seeds of rebellion begin to take root in your mind.

When your diet makes certain foods taboo, you may actually feel a heightened sense of excitement when you indulge in them, like you're doing something "naughty." You think, "Shhh, don't tell anyone, but I'm eating a cupcake!" and then you gobble it up and enjoy that rush of breaking the rules. Just like a recalcitrant teenager seeking a thrill, you rebel against the harsh restrictions of your diet and quickly return to all your bad habits. **Result: Failure.**

To keep you from staging a rebellion against this plan, I knew I couldn't strap you with mile-long lists of "no-no" foods that are strictly forbidden, because all you'd want to do is rebel anyway. Instead, I want you to know that losing weight does not require perfection or absolutes. No one can achieve perfection, and if you go in thinking that's the goal, you'll fail. What my plan requires is excellence. By that I mean that you're on track *most* of the time, not every second of every day. Yes, you must recognize that weight loss requires a willingness to change and an open mind. But it does not mean you must never again eat certain foods. In fact, I created a system for safe splurging on this plan, one that won't leave you feeling guilty. You're going to set a new pattern for yourself and the way you eat—but we're looking at a pattern across time. It's not the end of the world if you step outside the bounds a little every now and then, and because it's not, you won't automatically seek to rebel against the plan. **Result: Success.**

Impracticality and expense

When I pick up the newspaper and read a headline like, "Shocking Tragedy: Man Inexplicably Mauled by Pet Wolf, Raised from a Pup," I have to shake my head and wonder, "Did they really just use 'pet' and 'wolf' in the same sentence and it's 'shocking' the guy was attacked?" Come on, people. Wolves have been carnivorous predators for centuries, and some arrogant fool finds a wolf pup, raises it, teaches it tricks, and then one day he comes home a few minutes late, the wolf is famished, and suddenly the fool becomes dinner. Why? Because there is a tendency for all organisms to drift back to their norm. That wolf has deep-rooted instincts, and he's going to act on them when he deems it necessary.

We humans have core defining habits, values, beliefs, and behaviors that are also deeply entrenched. Sure, we can be pulled over to a new position, but we are going to start drifting back. Therefore, if your diet requires you to do something that is seriously divergent from your life pattern—if, all of a sudden, you can't eat with your family or go out to restaurants, you have to eat at odd times that don't fit your schedule, and so on—you are going to drift back to what is deeply entrenched. It's called "instinctual drift."

It's a concept that applies not just to what we eat, but also to exercise. In my case, for example, if you want to get me to exercise, ballet is not the way to go. That's so outside of my norm—I mean, can you see me in pointe shoes and a tutu? Not going to happen. But if you give me the option to compete in a sport involving a game and a ball of some sort, where someone's keeping score, now that appeals to my competitive nature and macho upbringing. That's where you need to meet me—on the tennis court—not in hot yoga or Pilates. Likewise, diets that force you far outside of your norm might work for a week, maybe two, but very quickly you are going to drift back into what you know.

Diets also don't work if they are so demanding that they seem to take over your busy life. If you're supposed to drink a special elixir the moment you wake up, memorize lists of what you can and can't eat, and then juggle Tupperware containers all day with "mini-meals" that you weighed and calculated, you might as well quit your day job, because your diet becomes practically a full-time job! Or maybe you're required to purchase expensive workout equipment (red flag) for a regimen that a US Army infantryman could barely follow! If a diet becomes an all-consuming obsession that doesn't fit into your already busting-at-the-seams (pun intended) life, it simply can't be sustained. **Result: Failure.**

If I'm going to prevent you from drifting back to the norm that's keeping you overweight and address this problem of impracticality, then I've got to give you a well-rounded plan that you can tailor to the flow of your life pattern. Look, I know your days move at a lightning pace—you're in a perpetual state of go, go, go and there still aren't enough hours to get it all done. You're not even sure if you locked the front door, much less if you added up all the fat grams in your breakfast correctly. So, I'm not going to give you impractical, time-consuming diet to-do lists that you can't sustain and that will cause you to rebel. Instead, I'll give you 30-second strategies, quick-prep meals, and even exercise routines that are fast and efficient so everything can be easily integrated into your agenda. I've also taken math out of the equation; on this plan, you don't have to add up calories, fat, sugar, carbs, or anything else. You'll learn by doing—eating the recommended meals and amounts of food in this plan can help you adapt to the right portions and recognize how much food you should be eating. The foods are easy to find and prepare, and you'll even know how to order when you're eating out.

But let me be clear: if you have fallen into a lifestyle pattern that is defined by food, if you truly live to eat, if you always have fattening foods at your fingertips, and you never break a sweat unless it's from reaching into the back of the pantry for your candy stash, well, your lifestyle is going to have to change. You have to be willing to make your health a priority. I'm not going to tell you that you can have your cake and eat it too. I'm simply saying this plan helps you effect positive change in a practical way.

This plan is also understandable and easy to follow; it's manageable even for your hectic life. But it will fly in the face of the permeating logic that the only way to lose weight is to eat next to nothing and avoid carbs (because they're the devil, right?). I'm going to tell you things that are easy to understand and implement, as well as provide you with information about new weight loss theories and emerging science to help you meet your weight loss goals. **Result: Success.**

Boredom

When you're eating the same exact foods day in and day out and your list of "safe" foods can fit very easily on a standard-size Post-it note, you're going to get bored. Monotony is certain death on a diet. If your diet consists solely of steamed chicken and celery, you quickly get to the point where you'd rather the damn chicken eat *you* than you eat another tasteless, dry hunk of white meat. Most people want variety, so if you deny your body that, you're steering the boat right into the storm. As your taste buds scream for something, *anything*, other than another bite of raw celery, you finally throw it down and make a beeline for the closest drive-thru window. And you know what else? A bland, boring diet does nothing to address your sugar withdrawal symptoms like we talked about before. So you feel bad, you're hungry, and you hate the foods on your diet. **Result: Failure.**

I understand that the moment you get bored on a diet is the moment that you start the downward spiral into failure, so this plan is designed to keep your taste buds engaged. I want you to look forward to eating and to enjoy the healthy foods your body needs, and you will be shocked by how quickly this can happen. Listen, if you've trained your brain to crave things like chicken-fried steak or ice cream sandwiches, you might not believe that you could ever crave something that's actually good for you. But because your body *needs* the nutritional building blocks found in fresh, whole foods, once you switch it into the mode of eating right, the shift will happen quickly. The meals on this plan are made with colorful, nutritionally dense foods and seasonings, rich in flavors and variety, so they check all the boxes and keep you from ever getting bored. **Result: Success.**

Temptations

If an alcoholic went to a rehab center that stocked every room with booze, how long do you think he'd stay sober? Come on, that's like asking a fish not to swim. When you're trying to lose weight and "sober up" from your long-running food addiction, your environment has got to prop you up and support your goals. Weight loss plans that don't address how to successfully set up all of your environments (I'm talking home, office, car, and your "virtual" environment) could be setting you up for failure. You simply don't stand a chance in moments of weakness when you open the freezer and there are cartons of ice cream and frozen pizzas staring back at you. **Result: Failure.**

I will show you how to program *all* of your environments for success. Again, when you are hungry, you *are going to eat.* So here's a novel thought: let's clean out your space so when it's legitimately time to reach for a snack, you aren't tempted with bags of chips lined up on the counter, a cookie jar, and nine boxes of popsicles. If you don't have all that available, then you've set up your world to support your "sobriety." The truth is, you don't *break* a bad habit; you must replace one behavior with a new one. And the new behavior should meet two criteria: it must be healthy, and it must be incompatible with the previous behavior.

That first criterion means you've got to replace the chips, cookies, and popsicles that you're removing from your environment with healthy alternatives that you actually enjoy eating. On this plan, you'll never, ever get caught with nothing to eat. You'll have the right foods available to you because as I've said, hungry people eat and they eat what is there, and you should *never* feel guilty about eating!

The second criterion means you need to adopt new habits that crowd out bad habits, because they cannot be done simultaneously. If you have a habit of coming in through the kitchen and consuming thousands of calories in "snacks" before you even take your jacket off, then let's figure out something that is incompatible with grazing around the kitchen. Go through the front door instead, or go directly to the gym right after work—do whatever it takes to get out of that old space, that old way of doing things, and into a new activity. I think you will be really surprised by how big of a role your environment is playing in your weight loss failure and how simple it will be to reprogram it so you set up habits to last you a lifetime. **Result: Success.**

Inconsistent results and plateaus

There you are, first thing in the morning, standing in front of the scale just hoping, praying, that all your hard work over the past week is going to pay off. You think about all the times you white-knuckled your way through cravings and fought off light-headed moments of sheer starvation, making for the world's longest month, and now, right now, you're going to see if it was all worth it. You squeeze your eyes closed, step on the scale, exhale, open your eyes and—WHAT?!—you *gained* a pound? How can this be? You followed that stupid diet chapter and verse! You turned down your grandma's apple pie at the family get-together and quit drinking soda cold turkey. This is an outrage! Impossible. Unthinkable. And, you're done. Diet is over. No payoff, no results right out of the gate—forget it. And then you wonder, "Is there any of that pie left?"

Or maybe a diet actually works for a little while but then suddenly you hit a screeching halt and the needle on the scale won't budge, no way no how. You've hit the dreaded plateau, which sends you into a tailspin, causing extreme frustration and destructive self-doubt. You start to think, "It's me. I'll never weigh one ounce less than I do right now. I might as well accept this fate, stop this insane diet, and go back to wearing muumuus full time and eating frosting straight from the container."

Whether it's the last five pounds or the last ten, if a diet doesn't offer a solution for getting over that hump, that diet is going out the window. And pretty soon, that muumuu looks like a minidress—it now goes sideways instead of down. **Result: Failure.**

If I'm going to keep you motivated, I know I have to be honest with you about weight loss. Experts indicate that you should aim for consistent weight loss of about one to two pounds per week, so you should remain realistic—you aren't going to lose 40 pounds per week (no matter what any diet product claims).

But I'll help you create healthy intermediate goals so that you feel good about what you're accomplishing along the way.

As for plateaus, part of the reason they occur is because when you're eating the same food and doing the same exercise day in and day out, you can get bored and lose motivation. That's why I've designed a plan with a number of exercises and numerous meals to help you stay interested and motivated. You should also restart the phases of the plan every 30 days to help introduce more variety into the plan. So, if you haven't reached your goal in the first 30 days of this plan, depending on how much more you have to lose, you will start over at one of the phases to continue your weight loss at a steady pace until you do hit your goal.

Plateaus can also strike when you're losing muscle mass on a diet, which happens when you're focusing solely on cardiovascular exercise and calorie restriction, as the majority of diets do! Muscles burn calories, and that's why I've incorporated a specific type of resistance training designed to build lean muscle tissue so that your body's caloric burn rate is amplified throughout the day. Even while you're sitting watching TV, your body will be working harder for you. **Result: Success.**

Like I said, I'm not the first person to come up with a diet that works, but I do know that by combatting the Top Seven "Ugly Truths" about Dieting, I've reverse-engineered a way to help you meet your weight loss goals. I want you to have 20/20 vision every step of the way. No surprises or gimmicky tricks, just a clear-cut, doable plan that gives you results. In the next chapter, we'll go over the basics of the plan so you know exactly what to expect.

2

A DIET THAT DEFIES
YOUR LOGIC

Status quo, you know, is Latin for "the mess we're in."
—Ronald Reagan

It's 8:00 a.m. in mid-March. You're in the bathroom getting ready for the day. You take one last look in the mirror, check all angles, and then you freeze. Your mind races: "What is *that*? Right there . . . that enormous bulge popping out over my waistband. Oh man, these pants used to be too big and now I'm spilling out all over the place." I know how you berate yourself, because you have told me a thousand times. You think, "This whole outfit makes me look like a giant stuffed sausage," or "Someone could seriously confuse me for the Michelin Man." I mean, did the dry cleaners shrink these clothes, or did I really pack on this many extra pounds over the winter? Just add it to my tab, right? Five pounds from work stress, 10 from the holidays, a few more from the visit with the in-laws—it adds up before you know it. Then you think, "I need to cut myself a little slack. It's been a tough few months. I just need to give up the double bacon cheeseburgers for a while and restart my gym membership, and then I'll be ready for swimsuit season in no time. Right?"

You've been telling yourself this same script again and again, year after year. And even if you did manage to cut back on junk food or drag yourself to the gym for a few sessions, has it ever worked in the past? I'm guessing the answer is no. But have you ever wondered why? It's what everyone says: you have to starve yourself and work out like crazy—isn't that the answer? New, developing research and theories suggest that the solution to your weight problem might go deeper than eating less and exercising more, though it's important not to under-emphasize the importance of healthy eating and exercise.

These theories and new research suggest that it's about the *types* of foods you're eating, the *kind* of exercise you're doing, and significantly, *how* you're changing your mindset and emotional responses. Let me give you an example. A 400-calorie low-fat blueberry muffin simply isn't capable of accomplishing the same things in your body as a 400-calorie bowl of oatmeal with apple slices and walnuts. They've got the same amount of calories, so you'd think they're "equal," right? Wrong. Way wrong. What you are going to learn in this diet is that not all calories are created equal, but the current research that's unfolding suggests that some foods may even have intrinsic abilities to help you lose weight, for example, by helping you feel full for longer.

I predict you are going to have a serious anger response when I give you the scoop on these new theories regarding what you need to eat and how you need to exercise in order to lose weight and keep it off with healthy lifelong habits. You are going to be thinking, "OMG! All this time, I never even had a chance! The miles I have walked around that damn track! The sacrifices I have made! The starvation I endured, the time I spent obsessing over what I ate, the pricey gimmicks—are you kidding me? I was dead in the water before I even started! I did it all with not even a chance of success."

This takes us back to the concept of using 20/20 hindsight to your advantage. I intend to completely revamp your current beliefs about weight loss, because that thinking hasn't worked for you, me, or anyone else. The latest theories based on new and evolving research are telling us that obesity is *not* reversed by cutting out carbs or fasting—both of which are methods you've probably tried before—but instead through the innate power of certain foods that could assist you in reaching your weight loss goals. My team of nutrition experts has identified the top 20 foods that this new research suggests may have specific effects on the human body to help weight loss. I refer to them as the 20/20 Foods.

The foods in this list each fall into one of three categories. Here they are:

Foods with Potential Thermogenic Properties

New theories suggest that some of the foods on this list can increase thermogenesis. "Thermo-what?" Well, thermogenesis is the metabolic process by which your body produces heat; in other words, it's related to your metabolism. There are different types of thermogenesis, and I'll explain more about that later in this chapter, but right now I'm specifically referring to "diet-induced thermogenesis." Some scientists believe that certain foods may increase your metabolism after you eat them. Did you ever think food could increase your metabolism? This is what I mean when I say that not all foods or calories are created equal.

Foods That Stick to Your Ribs

If you've ever sat down and polished off an entire family-size bag of nacho cheese chips at record speed and then felt hungrier than when you opened the bag, you know that not all foods you put in your mouth satisfy you.

But, believe it or not, there are also certain foods that research suggests may increase your satiety; they tell your brain that you've had enough and you don't need any more after eating a reasonable (not gargantuan) portion. They help you feel fuller than other foods in their same category—or, as we say in Texas, they really stick to your ribs. For instance, codfish and chicken are both lean proteins, but research indicates that people who eat cod report feeling fuller than people who eat chicken. I used this type of information to compile this list of filling foods. Think back to other skimpy diet meals you've eaten and how you've been left yearning for more. Maybe you even wound up in front of the open refrigerator, wiping drool from your chin, and then eating everything in there like a starving vulture. Well, the meals in this diet plan have been designed to help you leave the table feeling full and satisfied.

You might be thinking, "Yeah, feeling full right after my meals is great, but what about later when I'm running on empty again?" I know just how this goes: It's the first morning of your new diet and your paltry breakfast already seems like a distant memory, when all of a sudden, your stomach gives a little gurgle. Oh no. You try to ignore it but before too long, the gurgle has evolved into a full-on growl so loud that your boss heard it from across the office. You stare at the clock as each second feels like an eternity, your head begins to ache, and images of pastries begin to usurp all of your rational thoughts. It becomes a mental tug-of-war, and you know you'll never survive until lunch. You finally surrender and think, "Now, where did I stash those 'emergency' candy bars?"

This post-meal hunger scenario can lead to rebellion. So how do we address it it? Well, studies have revealed that certain foods have the particular ability to suppress your appetite, meaning they delay the return of your hunger so you can last until the next mealtime without having to seriously consider gnawing off your own arm. And because you're not hungry, you won't be haunted by cravings anymore.

I think what will really surprise you is that these are not the weird, unappetizing foods that can only be found at the pricey health food store. These also are not "fat-blasting" fad foods from some exotic rainforest somewhere. Examples include almonds, apples, and yogurt. Nothing crazy there! I want you to think of these as "everyday superfoods" that should be eaten in the right proportions.

Time–Release Combinations

The final method comes from new theories that suggest that foods should be combined to create a time-release type effect in your body.

These theories suggest that the right combination of carbohydrates (that's right—carbs are *not* the devil!), proteins, and what I call "fit fats" can cause your body to break meals down slower, and slower is better because it means your brain continues to receive the "full" signal for hours after you eat these meals. Plus, research suggests that eating these foods can help you feel more energized, which can help reduce the need to grab a sugary snack in the middle of the day for a pick-me-up. But the right portions are *really* important and the meals in this diet are designed with this in mind. By the end of the plan, you'll know how to combine foods and create appropriate portion sizes on your own so you can truly adopt this as an ongoing lifestyle.

Delicious, Flavorful Foods (No, Really!)

We've all heard the saying, "If it tastes good, spit it out." That's because if something tastes good, there's no way it could also be good for you, right? Because heaven forbid that a healthy meal could possibly be enjoyable or, oh, I don't know—have a little hint of flavor. How many diets have you done that had you eating foods with about as much flavor as Styrofoam? Most people equate "diet" with "bland" because that's always been their experience.

Just because you're losing weight doesn't mean you should have to dread every flavorless, predictable bite. Plus, there's a whole world of new information out there on the health benefits that various seasonings and herbs have to offer. Your body wants and needs these things, so why would you deprive yourself of them?

30-Second Strategies

This plan incorporates fascinating 30-second behavioral strategies to help you achieve your goals, and I think you will be amazed by what you can accomplish in just 30 short seconds with these. (And if you can't spare 30 seconds, then there are other problems we need to discuss first!) Furthermore, some of the meals can be assembled in 30 seconds, and even the exercise program is based on 30-second "bursts." Here's what it entails:

Exercise: Less Is More!

New theories suggest that long, drawn-out cardio sessions may not be necessary when it comes to weight loss and that shorter workouts of varied intensity may also be effective. There's lots of good news here: First, you don't need some kind of expensive equipment or membership at a state-of-the-art gym in order to perform this kind of exercise. Secondly, you may be able to exercise *less*, but still burn calories, making this exercise plan easy to fit into your schedule.

Don't get me wrong: you're going to be doing some work. If you're one of those people who leaves the gym looking like you just left the beauty salon, not a hair out of place and not a bead of sweat on your body, then you're not fooling anyone and you're wasting your time. But the secret to this exercise program lies within 30-second bursts of intense activity in between less intense activity. And if you hate running or can't run, don't worry: this method applies to biking, swimming, walking, or any other kind of exercise that floats your boat.

You'll learn all the ins and outs in chapter 10, but the bottom line is that this routine can help you lose weight, burn calories and fat, and tone shapely muscles—all in less time than you might imagine, and all in your own home.

Splurging Allowed (Yes, Even Alcohol)

"Cheat days" have become a trend in diets lately, but sticking to a plan for six days and then going completely bonkers at the all-you-can-eat pizza bar on day seven is going to get your body chemistry off kilter and you know it. So here's a concept: follow the plan every day, but know that you can have a reasonable splurge once or twice a week. Then you're not fixating on that day seven pig-out all week long, it doesn't take as much to satisfy your need for a little something that's "off plan," and it doesn't affect your steady weight loss.

After the first phase of this diet (which is only five days, by the way), you're allowed a splurge once or twice a week—this even includes a glass of wine. (In fact, some research suggests that some people who drink alcohol in moderation weigh less than people who don't!) There are some simple guidelines you'll follow to achieve fail-safe splurging: you'll ask yourself if you're really trying to fill an emotional need with food and, if so, address it in a different way; the splurge food must fit in the palm of your hand (I'll give you specific examples of splurge sizes so you don't overdo it); and you must do some form of exercise on days that you splurge.

Ultimately, this technique takes your focus *off* cheating because you know you are allowed to splurge, and in my experience, simply knowing that it's available means you actually end up splurging less often than you do on other, more restrictive plans.

Body Composition Overhaul

On a lot of popular diets, you may lose both fat *and* muscle because you're drastically restricting carbohydrates, which your muscles desperately need, and you're not exercising properly. Even if it reflects a lower number on the scale, you really do not want to lose muscle because it is the "furnace" that burns fat. Less muscle, smaller furnace. Smaller furnace, slower weight loss. But the meals in this diet are designed to allow you to maintain and build muscle.

Plus, with this plan we have provided a number of exercises that are easy to incorporate into your daily life that are designed to build muscle and help tone your body. So when you follow this exercise plan and lose 10 pounds, it might actually feel like 20 because the overall shape of your body is improving. You might even fit comfortably into clothing you wore when you weighed less. I know it seems strange, but your weight is not the whole story. Body composition is critical.

Getting in Tune with Your Hunger

Let's conduct a little experiment. Close your eyes and imagine biting into a crisp dill pickle. What happened? Come on, I can see you wiping the drool from here. Your mouth watered, of course! You began producing saliva in anticipation of eating a pickle. Maybe that doesn't seem like an earth-shattering revelation, but think about it: you didn't *see* a pickle, you didn't *touch* a pickle, you didn't *smell* a pickle; all you did was *think* about one.

Your thoughts have the ability to produce physiological responses in your body. In this plan, you're going to harness the power of your thoughts to help you lose weight instead of letting them run amok and contribute to the problem. One way you'll do that is by implementing my Hunger and Fullness Scale in your daily life. This scale will help you identify the difference between real, physical hunger, habit hunger, and that fake "mind hunger," which is just a feeling conjured by your thoughts, emotions, or responses to triggers.

Mind hunger is what happens when you succumb to either an external cue, like a candy jar or fast-food commercial, or an internal cue, such as stress or loneliness. It's not accompanied by physical symptoms of hunger like a growling stomach, which means your body does not actually need nourishment. The Hunger and Fullness Scale on page 71 will help you understand, based on signals your body is sending you, just how hungry you are so that you shouldn't get too hungry and you shouldn't eat when you don't actually *need* to. By getting in tune with your body and its signals, you will begin to gain control over your eating habits.

You've probably heard me say it before, and I'll say it again—you can't change what you don't acknowledge. Until you acknowledge that not all "hunger" means you must stuff something in your mouth immediately or risk passing out and dying from starvation, you can't have successful weight loss. I could throw every healthy food known to man at you, but if you haven't learned to pay attention to your body, and not overeat, you will remain overweight. And once you start paying attention, you will be shocked at how often you've been eating purely out of "mind hunger" or "habit hunger." It happens to everyone, but what sets you apart is that you're now identifying it and taking control over it.

Calling in the Experts

It's hard to lose weight if you *just* change your food, or *just* change your exercise, or *just* change your thinking. To be successful, we've got to tackle this from all angles. You have to shake it up to break it up. That's easier said than done and probably impossible to do alone. So, in order to give you a diet plan that addresses all of the "ugly truths" about other diets that have failed you, as I alluded to earlier in this chapter, I put together a top-notch team of experts across several fields.

If you have read any of my other books or watched me on TV, you know that my expertise is in the area of human behavior. I've been studying it and applying that knowledge with patients and guests on my show for four decades. And when it comes to weight loss, you might not immediately think of a psychologist as the type of expert from whom you would seek answers. Look, weight is a function of behavior, and your thoughts control your behavior. In a study published in the *Journal of the American Dietetic Association*, researchers found that subjects who ate out of stress or emotion were 13.38 times more likely to be overweight or obese. That's a huge number! Imagine how much better off you'd be if you could remove that emotional eating factor from the equation. This is exactly why I've got to help you stop using food for anything other than nutrition.

Here's the truth: even if you know exactly what it takes nutritionally and in terms of physical exercise to shed those pounds, putting it into action and sustaining it is the tough part. It's estimated that 80 percent of people who do succeed at losing weight will gain it all back. Why? Unless you alter your lifestyle and find new, nonfood ways to cope, you will eventually drift back to your previous behaviors. So I'm going to take what I know about human behavior to help you reprogram your thinking and your lifestyle so that they're designed to support your goals.

I've said for a long time that I wasn't going to write a new diet book until there was something new and intriguing enough to take the conversation to the next level. Well, when my research team and I sat down and really pulled apart this new information, I knew that time had come.

Food is, of course, a critical piece to this puzzle. A vital member of my nutrition team is registered dietician Cynthia Sass, who brings to the table a great deal of experience both with patients in her private practice and as a sought-after writer in the nutrition field. She's a *New York Times* best-selling author in her own right and has contributed to several well-known national health and wellness magazines over her career. With her bachelor's degree in nutrition/dietetics, her master's degree in nutrition science, and another master's degree in public health, Cynthia knows a thing or two about what, when, why, and in what combinations you need to eat food. And she has formal culinary training because she gets a vital point about all of this—you've got to *want* to eat the foods on your diet!

This plan is a 360-degree approach because I believe anything less will fail you. Now I'm going to show you just how all the pieces of the puzzle come together for you.

The Fly-By Version of the 20/20 Diet

This diet is divided into three phases over the course of 30 days. Here's a breakdown of each phase:

Overview of Phase 1: The 5-Day Boost

The first phase lasts a total of five days and helps your body find new dietary balance and restore itself. In these first, very important five days, you will build a momentum (a "boost") that will set you on a new path and keep you motivated. You will choose your meals and snacks (four a day, spaced about four hours apart) from a list of simple, delicious recipes that are created by using only the 20/20 Foods. The primary goal of this phase is to tune in to your body signals by learning how to distinguish between physical hunger, habit hunger, and mind hunger using my Hunger and Fullness Scale.

If your doctor OKs it, during this first phase you can also start the exciting (and fun!) 30-Second Burn Burst Exercise Program explained in chapter 10. If not, you will simply increase the number of steps you take throughout each day you're on this phase so you can prepare your body for more physical activity later.

Overview of Phase 2: The 5-Day Sustain

By the end of Phase 1, you'll be in a positive pattern of eating certain foods at specific times of the day, and your body and mind will be in a brand new groove. In the second phase, which is also just five days long, you'll continue to expand on your progress by introducing some new foods to the mix (no boredom here!). The primary goals of Phase 2 are:

- Start recognizing flavors better because the meal plans have been designed to rely on flavors other than added salt, sugar, and artificial sweeteners.

- **Splurge safely:** You won't be set up to rebel.

There's a new list of delicious meals to choose from so you don't have to think about how to combine foods in the correct proportions.

We're keeping it simple. Each meal will include at least two of the 20/20 Foods.

You'll also keep up the 30-Second Burn Burst Exercise Program or be walking more each day.

Overview of Phase 3: The 20-Day Attain

During these 20 days, you'll continue eating two of the 20/20 Foods in each of your four meals a day. The goals of Phase 3 are:

- **Maintain steady weight loss:** Keep losing weight and trimming inches.*

- **Dine out without slowing progress:** Apply simple strategies for dining in restaurants.

- **Discover variety:** Enjoy lots more foods and flavors to inspire healthy food preferences more than ever.

You'll find 80 meals to choose from (yes, you really could eat a different meal four times a day for all 20 days), and they're still combined for the right balance to fuel your body. Plus, you'll have a comprehensive list of options for what to order when you go out to restaurants.

Remember, everyone is different and we all lose weight at different rates, so maintain a realistic outlook on how much you're losing and how quickly.

The Power of the Right Portions and Proportions

In all the phases of this diet, we've designed each meal to have a certain amount of heart-healthy fats, lean protein, wholesome starches (also known as complex carbohydrates), and fruits/vegetables because the current findings suggest that the correct portions and combinations create thermogenesis and satiety.

Complex carbohydrates provide slow-burning energy and B vitamins. They are also your body's preferred fuel source, but in our plan we've created reasonable portion sizes that aid you with weight loss. Lean proteins help you burn calories in the hours after meals and maintain or build calorie-burning muscle. When you put these carbs and proteins together proportionally, the protein actually slows your rate of digestion of the healthy starches. That slower digestion means a better regulation of blood sugar and insulin levels, and your body receives its carbohydrate fuel in a time-released manner.

The right portions of "fit fats" may help you feel fuller for longer, support healthy circulation, and increase your body's ability to absorb key antioxidants and vitamins from your fruits and vegetables. Fats and proteins also provide the raw materials your body needs to support healthy bodily functions.

So, when you eat the meals that we've created every four hours, you know that your body is getting reasonable portion sizes of important nutrients to fuel you throughout the day. Like I said, we need to eat to live, not live to eat. And these foods will have you living a happy and healthy life.

Overview of the Management Phase

After 30 days, depending on how close you are to your goal, you may repeat the plan. When you've reached your goal weight, you'll begin the Management Phase of the diet. The goals of this ongoing phase are:

- **Help you adopt lifelong habits to make healthy weight a permanent part of your life.**
- **Solidify your new, healthy lifestyle.**

In this phase, you'll learn a simple formula for combining the right portions and proportions of foods in all of your meals. Again, it doesn't involve counting calories, doing math, weighing food, or anything complicated or annoying like that. It will simply help you strike the right balance between fats, proteins, starches, fruits, and vegetables while maintaining portion sizes to help keep you at your healthy weight.

The Role Your Metabolism Plays

Metabolism is a word that gets thrown around an awful lot these days, and as a result, you might have a misconception about what the heck it has to do with weight loss. It boils down to energy and calorie burning—it's all about how your body uses energy to support life, and that includes processes you don't think about but that still require energy. For example, you need energy in order to breathe, circulate blood in your veins and arteries, digest, think, heal, produce hormones, and so much more.

The energy your body requires to carry out those basic functions is called your basal metabolic rate, and it represents between 60 and 75 percent of the calories you burn on a daily basis. Everybody's basal metabolic rate differs. The number of calories you burn doing these basic processes of survival is based on your gender, age, and body composition.

Three Types of Thermogenesis

As I briefly introduced earlier, thermogenesis is the process by which warm-blooded animals like us regulate body temperature—it's our body's way of producing heat. Our bodies need energy in the form of food (calories) in order to stay warm, among many other bodily functions, and thermogenesis is how we use energy to produce that heat.

Thermogenic Source #1:
Non-Exercise Activity Thermogenesis (NEAT)

Normal everyday activity requires energy. For example, taking a shower, preparing food, working at a desk, and other unintentional exercise activity—those all require your body to burn calories too. These activities are referred to as NEAT, which stands for non-exercise activity thermogenesis. You can increase your NEAT by adding in simple, practically mindless movements while you're doing everyday activities. You'd be surprised how many more calories you can burn just by taking the stairs, parking farther away from the store, or standing up instead of sitting on your duff all day. It may not sound like much, but these little things add up in a big way.

Thermogenic Source #2: Exercise-Induced Thermogenesis

The next piece of the metabolism puzzle is exercise-induced thermogenesis—working up a good, old-fashioned sweat. This is the most obvious way in which your body burns up calories. It's cyclical: the more active you are, the more calories your body burns up in order to give you the energy for the activity. The 30-Second Burn Burst Exercise Program is a fun way to burn calories and is easy to fit into your lifestyle, so it's a win-win. No, I'm not asking you to go out and become a triathlete, but I am going to ask you to break a sweat.

Thermogenic Source #3: Diet-Induced Thermogenesis

The final aspect of metabolism is diet-induced thermogenesis. This is the process by which your body manages and digests the foods you give it. As we're learning from new theories, some foods may affect this process differently and help increase your thermogenesis after you eat them. In chapter 6, you will find information about these foods and the studies backing them.

Could You Be Weight-Loss Resistant?

My wife, Robin, has a great genetic metabolism. She could eat a flock of chickens, a sack of potatoes, and two éclairs and not gain an ounce. I am exactly the opposite. I have a genetically transmitted disorder called metabolic syndrome, or syndrome X. It is actually a cluster of conditions: high triglycerides, insulin resistance, and accumulation of lower belly fat. The insulin resistance means that many types of sugar and carbohydrates are like poison to my body and they can block my body's normal conversion of food into expendable energy. Instead, it stores it in fatty deposits. I am also diabetic, which further complicates my weight loss.

So I am predisposed to obesity—but I'm the only person in my family who is not obese. The reason is simple: they choose what they choose and I choose what I choose. I think I deserve to have a weight that allows me to have good health, longevity, activity, and a positive body image. I will not accept less from myself because I think I deserve better.

Am I a victim? No. If you are similarly situated, are you a victim? No. You just need to inform yourself, because this information affects your next steps.

If you think you fit into the weight loss resistant category, you should assess your weight loss needs with your doctor and let him or her determine the best course of action, as this plan may not be appropriate for your distinct medical needs.

Putting It All Together

In the next chapter, I'm going to introduce you to some of the psychological underpinnings of this entire plan. I want to show you how you can get out of your own way and stop sabotaging your weight loss efforts. Remember, there's no magic bullet that will make you thin in the blink of an eye. But by gaining control over your decisions, environment, and behaviors, you will shift how you look at food and exercise to make healthy eating and exercise a lifelong habit.

Even if you haven't seen your feet without sitting down for 20 years (yes, you can add that to your 20/20 vision of how your life will change), I'm going to show you that this is within the realm of possibility, and that you can achieve your goals if you truly are ready.

3

GETTING OUT OF
YOUR OWN WAY

We are what we repeatedly do. Excellence, then, is not an act, but a habit.
—Aristotle

When you look at those people whom you admire—maybe they're skinny, glamorous, seem to have it all—do you say to yourself, "They are better than me and I will never be able to look that way or feel the way they seem to feel. I guess I'll never have what they have; I've seen myself try and fail too many times." You may still feign excitement or get temporarily pumped up about some quick-fix fad diet, but deep down, do you really believe you can do it? If not, you won't do it.

If, on the other hand, you look at your role models and think, "Now it's my turn," then this is your chance to make it so. Listen, if you continue to do what you've always done, you will continue to have what you've always had. If you do different, you will have different. If you begin to require more of yourself, that in and of itself is *different*.

It starts by adjusting your thinking. You've got to abandon all your negative beliefs about yourself and replace them with positive ones. You have to identify and embrace what it is that you are good at, as well as the qualities, traits, and characteristics that make you a worthwhile human being.

I'll give you an example from my life. When I was a kid, my personal truth was severely damaged. My family was dirt poor, my father was a bad alcoholic, and there were even times growing up when I was hungry and homeless. I had to rally just to feel like a second-class citizen! But eventually, and with a lot of help from some coaches, I found something I could be proud of. As it turned out, I was a good athlete.

Now, obviously I was no Michael Jordan or Tom Brady, but on the football field, I could run pretty darn fast and jump pretty darn high and seemed to be able to catch and hang onto the ball better than most. Once that whistle blew, my team didn't care where I lived or who my family was; they cared that I could play football. And when I looked around to find that all of my teammates who I held in high esteem were suddenly deferential to *me*, they believed *I* was superior, I thought, "There must be something good about me because they're choosing team captain, and they choose me." So I focused on that one, isolated area, and that was enough for my self-worth to begin to grow.

Finding value in that one area gave me enough traction to stop putting myself down for what I *wasn't* blessed with and focus instead on what I *was* blessed with and worked hard doing. I was giving myself a fact-based attribution to my self-image.

You can do the same. There are four steps to get you started:

1. **Decide what you are good at or what is good about you.**

2. **Observe yourself exhibiting those qualities or characteristics or mastering a given function or activity.**

3. **Acknowledge that you are, in fact, living to your potential and having some mastery in your life.**

4. **Make an attribution to yourself regarding that competency.**

Now we need to apply this approach to how you feel about your body and losing weight. You've got to decide, and really believe, that you can be good at losing weight. As you learn to eat healthy and incorporate exercise into your daily routine, you will observe yourself mastering weight loss because the scale and the measuring tape will reflect that fact. You will change your personal truth to reflect the new reality you've created. And as your personal truth begins to change, you will stop beating yourself up for all the mistakes you've made in the past. Then you behave your way to success because once you've changed your thoughts and beliefs about yourself, your behavior follows.

Out with the Old

You need to begin this program with an open mind and a clean slate, not just about who you are but also about diet and exercise. Whatever you *think* you know about how to fuel your body and help it release the weight clearly hasn't worked for you so far, so we're going to introduce you to some new theories and tips that could help you succeed this time.

Perhaps you haven't been applying information you learned in the past correctly. For example, you heard once that a low-fat diet was the answer. So you bought every candy labeled "low-fat," ate the whole damn box, and then couldn't figure out why the pounds weren't melting away! You thought, "Hey, the packaging says it's a 'low-fat food' so I can eat the whole damn box!"

Well, guess what? Refined sugar, which is what that candy is made of, doesn't have any fat in it, but do you really think you could eat four pounds of it a day and not gain an ounce? Of course not! We now know that the excess sugar, or what's referred to as "simple carbohydrates," gets converted to fat once it's in your body, which translates to more pounds on the scale. You have to be armed with both the right information and the correct way to apply that information. Now we know better in so many areas that impact your body.

Right now, I want you to spend 30 seconds writing down all the ways you've tried to lose weight in the past. If you've tried fasting all week and then pigging out on the weekend, write that down. If you believe that the only way to get thin is to starve yourself, get that down on paper. If you've tried existing purely on sliced turkey and hamburger patties, add that to the list. Think of every diet, exercise program, system, cleanse, product, and procedure that you've tried and put them all down on paper.

Once they're in black and white, go through the list and cross out each one that has failed you. As you cross them out, I want you to acknowledge that these ideas did not work for you, but that you can still succeed in reaching your weight loss goals. Now, crumple up the paper and throw it away. Be as dramatic as you wish to drive the symbolism home; I don't care if you light it on fire (as long as you don't burn your house down!). The idea is that you're using your 20/20 hindsight to let go of the past, start fresh, and open your mind to the new information you're going to learn and master.

Your Mind/Body Connection

A powerful tool you should have in your weight loss arsenal is called guided imagery. Psychologists use this when working with cancer patients. They ask them to think of their disease as ants attacking them, or to picture their own immune cells as Pac-Man characters gobbling up all the cancer cells. This gives patients a sense of power and control over what can be a terrifying diagnosis. It also lowers stress and anxiety, alters brain waves, and has even been shown to increase the body's natural immunity. It helps patients dealing with serious illness, and it can also help you lose weight.

First, create a visual symbol for the extra fat on your body. It could be prison bars that are figuratively encasing and restricting you, or a black cloak with the hood pulled up, hiding you from others, or a massive python wrapped around your body, squeezing the life out of you. Then ask yourself: Why have you allowed this to happen? Why have you imprisoned yourself? Why are you hiding? Why have you given yourself a death sentence?

Your weight problem has likely been a gradual process, probably without conscious intent, but in most cases, arriving at this weight was *your* decision, even if it was a subconscious one, because there was some kind of payoff. You wouldn't have continued the behaviors that caused you to gain weight if there wasn't any payoff.

For example, victims of molestation sometimes make a subconscious choice to gain weight so they can feel sexually irrelevant and thus thwart all interest from the opposite sex, even healthy interest. Other people turn to food for pleasure, companionship, a sense of calm, a deep-seated need for immediate gratification, or an irrational form of reward. Your payoffs could be any or a combination of these factors, but the point is that you need to first recognize them and then learn how to generate the very same payoffs, except with healthy behaviors this time. I'll help you do just that as we continue working in the chapters ahead.

Now, go back to the symbol you've associated with your extra weight. Imagine yourself losing weight and as you do, see yourself overpowering, for example, that constricting snake so it's forced to loosen its grip on you, or watch as you bend those prison bars with superhuman strength, or as you peel off that heavy, black cloak. *You're* in control now. As you begin to lose weight in real life, return to this symbol over and over, until finally, the visual no longer applies at all.

Why Willpower Doesn't Work

A huge part of getting your thinking right is to understand the fundamental difference between "control" and "willpower." In our survey, we asked why people typically quit or gave up on weight loss programs. We gave a list of common reasons, including hunger, cravings, unsupportive friends and family, plateaus, and lack of willpower and asked respondents to rate the extent to which each issue affected their decision to throw in the towel.

Before I reveal the intriguing results, I want you to answer this question truthfully: If you've ever quit a diet or fallen off the weight loss wagon in the past, how much did your "lack of willpower" factor into your decision to quit? Use a scale of 1 to 10, where 1 means it did not play a role at all and 10 means it played an extreme role. If you answered "10," you are in good company. In our survey, 37.6 percent of people said "lack of willpower" was the top cause of their past weight loss failures. They gave it a score of 10 out of 10.

I've been saying it for years: willpower doesn't work long term. It's a temporary fix. You think, "This is it! I'm going to do it this time! I'm going to bulldoze my way through this and finally get skinny." Come on. You know how that story ends. You might manage to starve yourself for a few days, and maybe you even drop a couple pounds. But then what happens? All you think about are the foods you aren't allowed to eat until finally those thoughts give way to actions, that dam breaks, and you find yourself devouring a large pepperoni pizza without coming up for air. And then you blame yourself and decide you'll just have to muster up *more* willpower and it'll work the next time. And so the ugly, self-defeating cycle starts all over again.

I want you to wipe the concept of willpower from your vernacular and replace it with words and concepts like "control" and "programming."

Willpower has no staying power. Control and programming can last a lifetime because when you set up your world and your relationships to support your weight loss goal, you set yourself up for success that lasts. As you start implementing this plan in your life, you'll begin to take back control over your thoughts, your relationship with and understanding of food and nutrition, important aspects of your lifestyle and environment, and your commitment to exercise. And ultimately, I believe you'll win back control over your weight.

What's Your Excuse?

Let's talk about your typical, go-to excuse when you're trying to justify your bad behavior. When you've given yourself permission to eat a large pizza, the whole plate of fried mozzarella sticks, a ginormous

---

The Obesity Disease

The American Medical Association recently changed its definition of obesity from a "complex disorder" or a "chronic condition" to that of "disease requiring a range of medical interventions to advance obesity treatment and prevention." The medical experts are taking this threat to public health extremely seriously, and so should you.

While I'm at it, I'd like to give you a quick rundown of the top health conditions that the Centers for Disease Control and Prevention lists as caused or aggravated by obesity: coronary heart disease, stroke, high blood pressure, type 2 diabetes, cancers such as breast and colon, liver and gallbladder disease, sleep apnea, respiratory problems, degeneration of cartilage and bone (osteoporosis), reproductive health complications such as infertility, and mental health conditions.

Use your 20/20 foresight to think of your future self as you make this decision to take your health seriously.

---

soda, or any other variety of unhealthy food, how have you been justifying that self-defeating behavior?

I asked about people's justifications for overeating or indulging in unhealthy foods in the survey, and I'd like you to answer honestly too:

Rate the following justifications for overeating or indulging in unhealthy foods in terms of how frequently, commonly, or intensely you do it (where 1 = the least common/intense, and 10 = the most common/intense method). For example, if you constantly tell yourself you will burn off the extra calories, you might rate that justification as a 9 or 10, whereas if you only occasionally use that justification, you might give it a 2 or 3. Choose N/A for any options that do not apply to you.

I tell myself . . .	1	2	3	4	5	6	7	8	9	10	N/A
that I will burn off the extra calories	O	O	O	O	O	O	O	O	O	O	O
that if others around me can do it, so can I	O	O	O	O	O	O	O	O	O	O	O
that it was peer pressure	O	O	O	O	O	O	O	O	O	O	O
that it's worth it because it tastes good	O	O	O	O	O	O	O	O	O	O	O
to live in the moment; I'll do better tomorrow	O	O	O	O	O	O	O	O	O	O	O
that I'm hungry or that I physically need the food	O	O	O	O	O	O	O	O	O	O	O
that I can't afford healthier, fresh foods	O	O	O	O	O	O	O	O	O	O	O

The top three excuses people from our survey identified with the most were:

1. I tell myself to live in the moment; I'll do better tomorrow.
2. I tell myself it's worth it because it tastes good.
3. I tell myself I'm hungry and I physically need the food.

Take a moment to think about all the lies you've told yourself in the past, all the ways you gave yourself permission to engage in bad behavior. Isn't it amazing how easily you can cheat yourself out of the *right* choices by convincing yourself that you "deserve" the *wrong* ones? It's highly illogical when you think about it. You deserve a better life, you deserve better health, and you deserve to lose weight. But in the moment, you're reacting to a trigger, so you convince yourself that you "deserve" the pizza and beer. In your mind, you're calling it a reward when, in actuality, it is a punishment. You'll tell yourself something, *anything*, in order to make it OK for you to have momentary pleasure.

It's time to stop these self-defeating patterns. The next time you find yourself drooling over some ridiculously inappropriate food choice, take control of your thoughts. Replace the excuse to indulge with a rational thought from this list or one of your own so you have a clear-cut strategy when you have a moment of weakness:

- Choices I make now will impact my future. I will turn down this temptation now so that I don't regret my decision later.

- The payoff of instant gratification isn't enough for me anymore. I care too much about reaching my goals to sacrifice them for something that tastes good in a fleeting moment.

- If I'm genuinely experiencing physical hunger, I will eat something from this plan to hold me over until the next mealtime.

What's Your Routine?

If I asked you about your food routine, what would you say? Do you even have one? Or is eating more like a haphazard, "grab 'n' go," stuff something in your face when it's convenient scenario most days of the week?

Many of the overweight patients I've worked with and counseled over the years report that they pretty much eat whatever is around, whenever they can. But the *lack* of a purposeful routine is still a routine. It's not a healthy one and it's not one that lends itself to weight loss, but it's a routine nonetheless. And it actually could be a huge factor in your current weight problem, because the latest theories indicates that *when* (or how often) we eat is just as important as *what* we eat.

For one full day, write down everything that goes in your mouth. From the coffee with cream and sugar in the car to the handful of chocolate candies at work, the chicken nuggets you grabbed at the drive-thru to the bag of chips you inhaled while watching a sitcom; write it *all* down. You can record it in a food journal, in your phone, a spiral notebook, or a collection of Post-it notes. You should eat like you normally do on an average day; the only thing that's different is that you'll record it and keep that record.

To make this even more useful, you're also going to write down the time that you ate the foods and a little information about what you were thinking about when you ate them. If you weren't thinking at all, you can just write "nothing"—that's fine. Or if you ate as a response to hunger and all you were thinking about was that you were absolutely famished, write "famished." Alternatively, if you're thinking about how stressed out, pissed off, or exhausted you are, say so. All of it is very useful data.

This exercise is going to provide you with a world of information. It will reveal to you what kind of *value* you are assigning to your food currently. I'll get into that more later, but for right now, make a pact with yourself that, starting when you wake up tomorrow, you will record everything that you consume.

When the chart is filled in, look at your results. Do you notice a pattern? Are you coming to realize that more of your food choices are based on an emotion, a trigger, or just pure habit rather than a physical need to eat? Or did you let yourself get so hungry that by the time you finally ate, you severely overate?

My One-Day Food Journal		
Time of Day	**Food or Drink**	**What I'm Thinking About**

We're going to look at these habits and trends in more depth a little later, but for now, this is a great starting point for acknowledging your routine—one that we will change together.

Are You Ready? (Or Just Pretending?)

Do you want to be thinner but aren't willing to give up your favorite foods? You'd love to be healthier but exercise is out of the question? Are you still thinking, "I suppose I'll get around to losing weight at some point down the road"? If those thoughts ring true, then you are not ready and there is little or nothing that I can say to convince you to get ready at this point.

If, however, you have hit rock bottom and you know there is no option anymore, you are ready to throw out your old ways that weren't working and make immediate, necessary changes to achieve your goal.

Life rewards action. Stop thinking about losing weight and take action. Now is the time to get out of your chair and into the game, because life won't wait around for you to make up your mind.

In the next chapter, you will make a plan for achieving your goals and then, watch out world, you're on a mission and no one can stop you!

4

SET THE RIGHT GOAL

To map out a course of action and follow it to an end requires courage.
—RALPH WALDO EMERSON

Setting the right goal in the right way is imperative. In *The Ultimate Weight Solution*, I talked about defining your "get-real weight," and I coined that term for two reasons.

First, you have to get real about what is safe and achievable for you. If you're a six-foot-tall woman with broad, swimmer's shoulders and quadriceps thicker than most tree trunks and you want to weigh 125 pounds like all of your pint-sized friends, you would be setting an unrealistic, unhealthy, and likely unachievable goal weight.

You also have to get real about your target weight from a psychological perspective. You can't just pluck a number from thin air that you want to see on the scale because you'll set yourself right back on the loopty loop you know all too well. Think about your relationship with your body and set goals toward liking it, being proud of it, accepting it for all of your God-given uniqueness, and treating it with respect and love. You will experience a psychological shift in how you feel about your body as you go through the steps in this program.

Watch Your Transformation

People are posting selfies all over the Internet these days, but I'm asking you to take a selfie that is for your eyes only. We already know how powerful it can be to look at the past, and we know you've got to clearly envision all that lies ahead. Now let's create markers to help you track your progress and pave your route.

Take a "before" photo of yourself when you start this plan, and then take photos at the end of each week so that you can watch the physical transformation occurring. You see yourself in the mirror every day, which can make it easy to miss physical changes, so that's where the photos come in very handy for continued motivation.

Also, take some simple starting measurements. Stand up straight and don't suck in or push out your stomach; just keep it neutral. Don't flex your muscles either. You want to get an accurate, neutral reading for all of these. As you progress through the plan, take the same measurements and record them in the chart below to help you track your progress and keep you motivated. You'll likely notice an improvement overall in muscle tone and your physical shape.

The point is not to obsess over these numbers. Again, these are simply opportunities to gauge your progress and pat yourself on the back as you feel pride over creating positive results.

	Starting Measurements	After Phase 1	After Phase 2	After Phase 3
Weight in pounds				
Around waist at belly button				
Around lower abdomen (just above hips)				
Around hips at widest area				
Around widest part of upper arms				
Around widest part of thighs				

Waist Circumference Warning

Quite a bit of research has been done in the area of measuring risk factors for cardiometabolic diseases such as diabetes, hypertension, and coronary heart disease, and one very simple way to determine your own risk is to look at your waist measurement.

In general, if you are a woman and your waist circumference is greater than 35 inches around, or if you're a man and it's greater than 40 inches around, then you are at an increased risk for serious illnesses.

Why? Well, your waist measurement is an indication of the amount of visceral fat in your body, and when I say visceral, I'm referring to the fat underneath your abdominal wall. This is the dangerous fat surrounding and in a sense "strangling" your organs and keeping them from functioning properly. This stuff is no joke—if you have this excess belly fat, and your measurements are in the danger zone, I want to sound the alarm loud and clear. And I want you to get serious about losing weight, so run, not walk, to your doctor to discuss what steps you need to take to reduce your risks.

The last step in this process of setting your sights on a clear target is to look at the chart on the next page and find your healthy weight range. Now again, this isn't a perfect science, but these weight ranges are typically considered within the realm of healthy for their corresponding heights.

Of course there are exceptions. Some people are long and lean, while others are naturally stocky. While some body types put on muscle very quickly, others just aren't designed to show muscle definition. You do have to use common sense and set a goal that is realistic. If you feel you are at a healthy weight, but fall outside of the range below, I recommend you talk to your doctor to help assess your weight needs.

Use this table to set your sights on a goal that is reasonable for *your* body.

Height	Ideal Weight Range
4' 6"	77–103 lbs.
4' 7"	80–107 lbs.
4' 8"	83–111 lbs.
4' 9"	86–115 lbs.
4' 10"	89–119 lbs.
4' 11"	92–123 lbs.
5' 0"	95–128 lbs.
5' 1"	98–132 lbs.
5' 2"	101–136 lbs.
5' 3"	104–141 lbs.
5' 4"	108–145 lbs.
5' 5"	111–150 lbs.
5' 6"	115–154 lbs.
5' 7"	118–159 lbs.
5' 8"	122–164 lbs.
5' 9"	125–169 lbs.
5' 10"	129–174 lbs.
5' 11"	133–179 lbs.
6' 0"	136–184 lbs.
6' 1"	140–189 lbs.
6' 2"	144–194 lbs.
6' 3"	148–199 lbs.
6' 4"	152–205 lbs.
6' 5"	156–210 lbs.
6' 6"	160–215 lbs.
6' 7"	164–221 lbs.
6' 8"	168–227 lbs.

Your 20/20 Vision of Your Future Self

An important aspect of goal setting has to do with defining the types of improvements you'll be making and how your life will change. Answer these questions honestly:

On a scale of 1 to 10 (where 1 = not at all and 10 = extremely), rate how your weight has affected (or is currently affecting) your:

	1	2	3	4	5	6	7	8	9	10
Sex life	O	O	O	O	O	O	O	O	O	O
Social life	O	O	O	O	O	O	O	O	O	O
Romantic relationship(s)	O	O	O	O	O	O	O	O	O	O
Work/Professional life	O	O	O	O	O	O	O	O	O	O
Non–romantic relationships	O	O	O	O	O	O	O	O	O	O
Ability to participate in physical activities	O	O	O	O	O	O	O	O	O	O

I'm guessing your answers revealed that your current weight is impacting most, if not all, aspects of your life. Now, let's dig a little deeper. Write down exactly what you've *wanted* to do that your weight has *restricted* you from doing. These are the aspirations that you've put so far on the back burner that you've nearly forgotten them. You must be *realistic* so you don't set yourself up for disappointment. If your "dream" has been to pose on the cover of the *Sports Illustrated* Swimsuit Issue, you might need a reality check. But maybe you want to strike a sexy pose in your bikini on the beach this summer? Now we're talking.

Here are a few more ideas to get you thinking: Maybe you want to set a goal of getting back into the dating world after years of keeping to yourself out of embarrassment. Or perhaps you want to fit into rides at the amusement park when you go with your kids, or simply fit into your favorite pair of jeans that you buried in the back of your closet.

Write down your dreams and goals below.

Part 1: What I Want to Do

....

....

....

Part 2 of the exercise is to spend at least 30 seconds visualizing yourself actually *doing* these things. This will allow you to *see* your own potential even before you've reached it. Athletes do this all the time. As basketball players stand at the free-throw line, they vividly see themselves in their mind's eye shooting the ball and the ball landing in the basket. Nothing but net! Golfers "watch" the ball go in the hole before they make the putt. I want you to program your mind by capturing a specific mental image not only of you doing these things, but what you will look like, what you will feel like, and how your life will be different after you've broken free of the bonds of being overweight. Imagine those feelings of passion, excitement, or whatever it may be for you and then imprint them in your mind. It's a step toward behaving in a way that will make it a reality.

When you're finished with the visualization, write it down.

Part 2: How I Will Feel

....

....

....

That might have been an emotional experience, especially if you've been afraid to let yourself think about what "could be" instead of wallowing in what "is." Maybe you've been blocked by fear of failure, or a fear of getting carried away in a dream that can never be your reality. I want you to claim victory over fear right here and now. This time, you will not fail. This time, it's within your grasp.

Create Your 20/20 Plan

Now let's create your plan to reach your goals. This is a process that I've been using and recommending for years because I've seen it work with people I have counseled. It gives you the ability to program yourself for success.

In short, the steps are:

- Express your goals in measurable and realistic terms.
- Express your goals in terms of specific behaviors and feelings.
- Assign a timeline to your goals.
- Break down your goals into manageable steps.
- Create accountability.

We'll go through each one together.

Express Your Goal in Terms That Can Be Measured and Are Realistic

Too many folks make the mistake of starting a new weight loss regimen with the unclear, unquantifiable declaration of "I want to lose weight." That is a wishy-washy, loose, weak statement made by someone who isn't serious about what lies ahead. If all you're saying is you want to lose weight, how will you know when you've reached that goal? When you've lost one pound? Ten? You won't know because you haven't stated it in a measurable way. A winner, someone who is programming himself or herself for success, states his or her goal with great specificity. Your weight loss goal must be measurable and realistic.

If you are 20 pounds overweight, then you would express your goal by writing, "I intend to lose 20 pounds to reach my goal weight of 130 pounds." Or if you choose to focus on your waist measurement instead of your weight, your goal might be expressed as, "I intend to lose 3 inches around my waist to reach my goal waist circumference of 34 inches."

My Measurable, Realistic Goal(s) Are:

....

....

....

Express Your Goal in Terms of Specific Behaviors

You behave your way to success. So, you have to get specific about what behaviors you will need to start doing, stop doing, or continue doing in order to achieve your goal. For instance, you might need to stop eating fast food and start doing the nutrition plan described in this book. Or you might need to shuffle your daily schedule to accommodate exercise, or get a physical activity tracking device so you'll move and walk more every day. You might need to continue doing meditation because it's reducing stress in your life.

I can't emphasize enough how important your past mistakes are here. You already know what hasn't worked, so add those routines and self-defeating behaviors to the lines below. Search all areas of your life for what you should stop, start, or continue doing in order to help you reach your goal.

I Need to		
STOP Doing:	*START Doing:*	*CONTINUE Doing:*

Assign a Timeline to Your Goal

The difference between a goal and a dream is a timeline. If you start this program with the attitude of "I'll lose weight someday," I can almost promise failure. "Someday" is not a day of the week. So, pull out the calendar and assign a realistic timeline to your goal. This is exciting because you will literally mark a day in your future, and that is the day you will have reached your goal (if not sooner).

Notice I said your timeline needs to be *realistic*. If you're still off in la-la land thinking you will be bikini-ready in three weeks even though you have 20 pounds to lose, you're kidding yourself. A realistic amount of time to lose 20 pounds is between 10 and 20 weeks.

You should also set incremental goals to help you maintain motivation. Rather than setting a date for when you'll achieve your final goal, give yourself some mileposts along the way. If you want to lose six pounds in the first month, write that down, and then when you achieve it, attribute that success to yourself so you can see yourself being successful at losing weight. This will help you define your personal truth as a winner.

Below, clearly state your weight loss goals in terms of a timeline. You can break it down week by week; whatever is going to work best for you. But write it here and set alarms in your smartphone or add it to your desktop calendar so that you have visible reminders. (Have you noticed yet how important a role I think vision plays in your success?)

My Realistic Timeline/Incremental Goals

....

....

....

Break Down Your Goal into Manageable Steps

Next, you need to define precisely what steps you're going to take in order to achieve your goal. You may not know every single step you'll need to take just yet, and that's OK. This list should evolve with you throughout the program. As you learn what is required of you, come back and add to this list.

For now, the steps might be more general, such as "I will learn and apply the information in this book," or "I will resolve to get up at least once per hour and walk around," or "I will stop going to the drive-thru."

The Steps I'll Take to Reach My Goal

....

....

....

Create Accountability

Next, you need to identify someone, or several people, to whom you can be accountable. You should tell them about your goal, your timeline for achieving it, and the steps you're taking so that you can check in with them on a weekly basis and update them on how you're progressing.

You should also feel comfortable enough with the person or people that you can call on them if you're feeling frustrated or if you want to share and celebrate milestones along the way. This can be a trusted friend, a family member, a spouse, or anyone close to you.

Below, list the person or people to whom you will be accountable:

My Partner(s) in Accountability

....

....

....

Congratulations on creating this imperative strategy for identifying and reaching your goal. *Knowing* what you want is the first step toward *getting* what you want, and it creates a positive momentum toward making it real. You're making some serious headway.

Imagine a scenario with me. You're sitting in a room, and this room has wall-to-wall zebra rugs, a zebra-stripe pattern on every inch of wallpaper and on every chair, there are photos of zebras on the wall, sounds of the Serengeti are playing in the room, and when you look out the window, a herd of zebras walk by. Literally all of your senses are being bombarded with a zebra message.

And then imagine that I ask you to think about something, anything . . . except zebras. What are you going to think about? If you didn't say zebras, you're not paying attention! It would take a lot of concentration and blocking out of your immediate surroundings in order to think about something other than a four-legged animal with black and white stripes.

That is an abundantly obvious example, but let me ask you this: If all of your senses were being saturated with images and smells of all the crap foods that led to your weight gain, why *would* you do anything other than think about them, salivate over them, and ultimately eat them? Asking yourself not to eat junk food when you are surrounded by it is practically a form of torture.

Overweight people, as a general rule, tend to be externally controlled—more so than people of average weight. For example, if two groups of people, one overweight and one of average weight, were served lunch that clearly wasn't enough food, but they were told there was more food in the fridge if they wanted it, which group do you think would go and get more food? The answer might surprise you. The people of average weight are more likely to get more food because they hadn't had enough to feel satisfied. They are controlled by internal stimuli, physical hunger. Because the overweight group is externally controlled, they eat what is there and stop. They likely wouldn't seek more from the fridge. But if the two groups were served a massive amount of food (think "family style" meal), who is more likely to continue eating until every plate is licked clean? The overweight group, because they see the food in front of them and so they continue to eat way past the point of being full.

Many of the decisions you're making about what you eat probably have to do with reactions to some kind of external stimuli. You see the candy in the jar on the counter, and even though you weren't thinking about candy—you weren't even thinking about *eating* (since you weren't experiencing physical hunger)—what do you do? You open the jar, grab a handful, and pop it in your mouth—maybe without even realizing you did it. You reacted to a visual stimulus. It's as basic as that. And the fix is just as basic. Remove the stimulus and replace it with a healthy alternative.

Notice I said remove it *and* replace it. It's not enough just to clear the house out of all junk food because eventually you are going to get hungry, and when you do, if there's literally nothing to eat except a jar of year-old pickles and some stale crackers, you're probably going to return to old habits and hit the drive-thru or order a pizza. Instead, you have to replace the unhealthy choices with healthy ones.

Listen, I can cure obesity, smoking, and alcoholism with 100 percent efficiency. No kidding! If you're smoking four packs a day and I parachute you into the Antarctic with no tobacco, guess what? You're cured. Right? Control the environment and you can eliminate these problems. If you don't have access to the substance, you can't abuse it.

The reason food addiction is more difficult to manage than alcohol or smoking is because you *must* interact with food. You don't ever have to interact again with alcohol or tobacco, but food—well, it's pretty basic for survival. But you can still program your environment so you don't rely on emotions for your food decisions. If you wake up in the middle of the night craving potato chips, it's pretty hard to give in and eat them if they're not there. Sure, you could get up, get dressed, drive down to the convenience store, and buy some, but that's a lot harder than just walking into the kitchen and bingeing. So you've got to set up your environment so in those moments when you don't feel strong, or your commitment is waning, your environment props you up.

Since I first discussed the concept of a "no-fail environment" in *The Ultimate Weight Solution*, the definition of "environment" has expanded significantly. Sure, you still live, work, and play in physical spaces. But as technology has exploded and become more readily available to an enormous cross section of society, our "space" now extends to cyberspace. Think of all the millions of times you might be exposed to messages relating to food: in e-mail, on social media, when surfing the web, and so on. Whether it's in the form of online advertising or friends posting images of their colossal dessert, it can be overwhelming. There's even a trend called "food porn" where people apparently post photos of drool-worthy foods online. Not to mention what you're watching on TV, looking at on your e-reader, or staring at in magazines! Our society is food obsessed, but *you* don't have to be.

So, let's investigate all the areas of your life that are crying out for you to convert to no-fail environments. The first step is to identify your cues. What are your "candy jar on the counter" stimuli? Here are some examples of cues that might often cause you to eat even when you are not physically hungry:

Common Food Cues

- Fast-food restaurants along your common routes
- Cooking or food-centered TV shows
- Images of food on social media/photo-sharing sites
- TV and Internet commercials
- Vending machines
- Seeing foods in the fridge, freezer, pantry, etc.
- Billboards advertising restaurants or foods
- Magazine advertisements
- Certain foods or drinks that typically cause cravings
- Smells of food emanating from restaurants
- Birthday parties or gatherings of any kind
- Being in places where you have typically allowed yourself to "pig out" in the past

Some or all of these may apply to you, or you might have other cues. Take a moment to analyze your own external food cues. Of course you cannot remove every single cue from your life. There are, however, many simple changes you can make to reduce the number of cues you experience on a daily basis. The most obvious one is clearing your kitchen of processed junk foods like chips, candy, soda, white bread, sugary cereal, pastries—you get the point! If it's something that will call out your name and tempt you to the point of you losing control, then it needs to go.

I've always said, the McGraw men are tough: we can handle anything except pain and temptation. Sound familiar? It's OK—most people are that way. If something hurts, they quit. If something's available, they start. So if you go home and your environment is chock-full of your personal poison, you are going to fail. This is why I don't recommend alcoholics go get jobs as bartenders. I mean, come on. Even Homer Simpson could figure that one out! Isn't the same true for you? If you are a recovering obesity patient or just looking to achieve a healthy weight, we don't need you going into (or living in) a target-rich impulse food environment.

This extends outside your home too. If there's a fast-food joint you pass on the way to work every day and it instantly puts you in a state of milkshake dreams, you might need to find a new route, even if it adds a few minutes to your commute. Or you might need to remove a friend from your social media accounts if he or she constantly tempts you with food references. Hey, it's nothing against her. Instead, add people who enhance what you're doing by posting their exercise routines or giving healthy ideas for meals. And if you're "addicted" to the latest show about decadent foods but by the final credits you've consumed approximately 10,000 empty calories, it might be time to install parental controls on that TV to keep *yourself* from tuning in. So I'm asking you to identify your external food cues, and then come up with ways to reduce your exposure to them.

In the next chapter, you'll find a clear list of foods with which you should stock your kitchen so that you have the right options to reach for when your stomach starts growling. As we know, hungry people will eventually eat (as they should!), and I want you to be prepared with the *right* foods.

"But What Will My Kids Eat?"

If you're worried about clearing out the kitchen of all the crap and thinking, "My kids aren't on a diet; I can't expect them to give up their favorites and eat this healthy stuff," this is my response: That is a higher form of parental insanity. You weren't born craving high-fat, high-sugar junk food. Your palate has *learned* to crave those foods. So now you're going to start training your kids' palates by gorging them with high-fat, high-sugar, and high-sodium foods so that becomes the norm for them too? If you do that, you're setting them up for complete failure.

As our country's obesity crisis grows, kids are anything but excluded. In fact, according to the Centers for Disease Control and Prevention, in the past three decades, childhood obesity has doubled and obesity in adolescents has more than *tripled*. More than one third of the kids in this country are overweight or obese. To me, that's just a tragedy. And of the overweight or obese children, 80 percent of them grow up to be overweight and obese adults. Why don't you take a guess at how much that costs us in additional medical costs? The answer is $190 billion.

I want to make you urgently aware of the fact that you are imprinting in your children's minds what their relationship with food should resemble, and you are setting up habits for them that they will carry through the *rest of their lives*. Twenty years from now, do you want them to be in the same boat you are right now? Do you want them to struggle with their weight, suffer through bullying, or even get diagnosed with a life-threatening disease? Of course not! You don't let your kids sit around and smoke cigarettes all day, do you? So why would you feed them what amounts to poison on a daily basis? If you teach your kids to choose a bowl of berries for dessert instead of an enormous ice cream sundae, that's a pattern they will continue to follow. Your job is to prepare your child for the next level of life, so let's not trick them into liking foods that could harm them.

continues ▶

So while you're changing your own decisions about food, take steps to get your kids on the healthy bandwagon too. I know, I know—taking away all the junk at once might lead to a meltdown of epic proportions. It's OK to keep a few snacks in a "kid cupboard" that is only for them, but limit their intake to one serving per day. And work with them to stock the kitchen with healthy alternatives they'll eat and enjoy the rest of the time. Of course, your kids are going to have cake and ice cream at birthday parties and some candy on Halloween—I'm not suggesting you go to extremes here. But just like you, once healthy eating becomes the status quo, you'll find that they'll stop constantly begging for junk food and start craving and asking for healthier foods before you know it.

Claim What's Yours

As you begin this diet, I want you to step way out of your comfort zone and audaciously claim what can and should be yours. Maybe you feel like you've spent your entire life focusing your attention on the needs of others, taking care of everybody else, and as a result, you've ended up with a list of priorities that doesn't include your own health or well-being.

I want you to claim your goal weight, your renewed health, and your brand new life right now. Know, and I mean really know, that you are capable of this, that you deserve it, that you're up to this challenge (and it *will* be challenging at times). If you get on task about this and you make this your top priority, your weight will no longer be a problem. You've got to name it to claim it.

20/20 Preparatory Exercises

Here are some quick steps you can take to ensure that you're all set and ready to start attaining your weight loss goal. These should take about 30 seconds each to complete:

Environmental Audit: Perform a mental audit of all your various environments. Have you adequately transformed them into "no-fail" environments?

Realistic Role Model: Think of a role model in the health/wellness realm you wish to emulate. Pick someone who is realistic and who promotes healthy philosophies. This person can help inspire you through your journey.

Make a Date with the Grocery Store: Pull out your calendar and schedule a trip to the grocery store to purchase the 20/20 Foods before you begin Phase 1. Important: Go to the store *after* a meal so you're not hungry and drooling over the junk food.

Contract with Yourself

You have already identified someone to whom you can be accountable for staying on the course toward your goal. But the most important person to whom you are accountable is *you*.

All I'm asking you to do right now is to set it in stone with the contract found on the next page. This is a visual symbol of the commitment you are making.

My Commitment Contract

I, _____ (your name), commit to follow the steps and timeline I have laid out in order to achieve my realistic weight loss goals. Just as in life, this diet is not going to be a success-only journey. Therefore, if I deviate along the way, I promise not to beat myself up or use it as an excuse to fail. Instead, I will get right back on track. I promise not to make excuses or to sabotage myself or allow others to sabotage my efforts. I recognize that I am in control of my decisions. I believe in my ability to use 20/20 foresight to achieve my goals, and I believe I deserve better for myself.

Signed,

_____   _____
(signature)   (date)

5

EXTINGUISH YOUR
FAKE HUNGER

Statistics show that of those who contract the habit of eating, very few survive.
—GEORGE BERNARD SHAW

Hunger is a gift. That's right; hunger, defined as the sensation you get when your empty stomach alerts your brain that you need food, is a gift. Hunger helps you stay alive. The need for food, which is our source of energy, is one of our basic survival needs, and it is the gift of hunger that tells us when we *need* food.

You get into trouble when you ignore your body's signals or start putting food in your mouth when the hunger sirens haven't yet sounded. I want to show you how to tune back in and stop misusing (and abusing) food.

I used to carry around a pocketknife all the time. Someone would ask me to borrow it and my first question was, "What do you plan to use it for?" I wanted to know because if they wanted to use it as a screwdriver, to pry at something, or for anything *other* than cutting, then the answer was "no." That blade is meant for one thing and one thing only: cutting. If you do something else with it, you'll break the blade right off. Like my pocketknife, you can't use food for anything other than its intended purpose. (Well, you can, obviously, but you will have to pay the consequences if you do.) Instead, we need to work together to change your behaviors.

Now, this doesn't mean you can't enjoy the taste, texture, and sensation of eating. You can still appreciate food. But ultimately the purpose of eating needs to be for nourishing your body, not fulfilling another need or desire. If I can get you to stop misusing food, then we're good. But your mind has likely learned that food is its go-to salve. Think about it. Feeling sad? Let's eat. Lonely? Got to eat. Time to celebrate? Bring on the food. No date tonight? That's OK, order a pizza. It's pretty outrageous when you think about how practically everything we do and every emotion we feel leads to some form of eating. I mean, we're like horses walking around with feedbags attached to our faces—it seems like we, as a society, are constantly *eating!* Heck, we've even trained our pets to go against their instincts and misuse food—just look at all the fat dogs and cats these days.

In order to "stop the madness," control your habits, and overcome impulses, you have to relearn how to identify your hunger signals and recognize the different types of hunger you're experiencing. We touched upon this earlier, but let's dig in a bit more.

First, there's physical hunger, which brings about physiological symptoms, like a growling stomach, or if you've really gone too long without eating, you might get headaches, dizziness, or become light-headed. And, of course, there are levels of this physical hunger, a range between a tad "peckish" and ravenous enough to swallow a cow whole.

Then there's what I refer to as "mind hunger," which is that feeling you get when you experience an emotion that you've been fixing with food. That's the one you've probably been responding to without even realizing it. For example, if you typically eat when you're stressed at work, then the next time the boss yells at you, you might experience a twinge of hunger, urging you to stop by the vending machine on the way back to your desk. It's not that your body actually *needs* food in order to continue functioning in that moment; instead, you have inadvertently trained your brain to signal you to eat under certain circumstances. It's a physical response to an emotional need. Sometimes you might even convince yourself that you're experiencing hunger, when you're really experiencing a trigger-induced craving.

Finally, there is also what I refer to as "habit hunger," which is an environmental or situational hunger response. You might eat because it's "time to eat," or because you're in a place where you typically eat, or you're doing something you have often paired with food, such as watching a movie or the Super Bowl, or taking a long drive.

To help you regain a normal, healthy perspective on when and how much to eat, I have developed my 20/20 Hunger and Fullness Scale. I want you to study this scale and start using it before you eat so that you can determine if you're physically hungry or if you're experiencing mind hunger or habit hunger. As I said, there are true, physical symptoms associated with hunger. It might have been a long time since you actually went long enough without food to feel this way. This is an incredibly useful tool that I want you to use every day until you really get it down.

Dr. Phil's 20/20 Hunger and Fullness Scale

1—Weak, unable to concentrate, hunger headache.

2—Extremely hungry, stomach growling nonstop.

3—Normal hunger, a little stomach growling, need to eat soon, but not ravenous.

4—Food sounds good, but not experiencing physical signs of needing food like growling stomach.

5—Not hungry but not full either—neutral.

6—Satisfied but not too full. Pleasant.

Ideal Range (left margin) *Ideal Range* (right margin)

7—Full, a little too full. You know you could have eaten less.

8—Too full, feeling stuffed, a little uncomfortable.

9—Experiencing more physical signs of eating too much: bloated stomach, sleepy, quite uncomfortable.

10—So full you're sick, nauseated, miserable.

How to Use the Hunger and Fullness Scale

Before you start each meal, you should be right at a 3. And you shouldn't let yourself fall beneath a 3 under any circumstances. Going too low on the scale could put you in danger of a major binge session. I'm talking double meat, double cheese, with a heaping helping of diet failure.

That's one of the biggest mistakes folks make when they're dieting—they think that they have to starve themselves, so they walk around with their stomach going, "Hey, dummy, I'm running on 'E' down here! Fill 'er up!" until finally they just give in and eat anything (and everything) in sight. When you deprive yourself of nutrition, your body will switch into "survival mode" and begin holding on to fat deposits. It's your body's way of keeping you alive when there's no fuel coming in. That's great if you're lost out in the wilderness and starving, but not if you're trying to lose weight.

In the first few days of Phase 1, if you find yourself dropping below a 3 an hour or two before mealtime, you can snack on a handful of almonds, walnuts, or pistachios to get you over the hump. The goal here is to eat only enough to take the edge off so that you're still at a 3 when it's time for your next meal. Keep a stash of these three types of nuts with you so you're not tempted by fast food or vending machines when you're away from home. Just don't overdo it—a handful of nuts (not a one-pound bag) has enough fat, protein, and calories to satiate your hunger for a while.

On the other end of the scale, instead of getting all the way to a 9 or 10 at mealtime, put the fork down when you reach a 6, even if there's still food on your plate. Now, maybe you were raised in a time or a home where food was scarce and you developed the mindset of "eat it when you've got it," or the directive to "clean your plate" is so ingrained in you from childhood that you can practically hear your mother's voice when you sit down at the table.

I wanted some insight into just how your upbringing might have shaped your current eating habits and relationship with food, so I asked about it in our national survey. Go ahead and answer this question, and then I'll show you how you compare to the national sample.

When you were growing up, did your family (check all that apply):

☐ Have healthy eating habits (encouraged fresh fruits, vegetables, lean protein sources)

☐ Have unhealthy eating habits (served primarily junk food, fried most foods, had little or no emphasis on fresh, whole foods)

- ☐ Equate food with love (e.g., "I cooked your favorite meal.")
- ☐ Keep the kitchen stocked with processed or junk food (e.g., soda, chips, cookies, pastries)
- ☐ Reward you with food (e.g., candy for good grades, dessert for finishing meal)
- ☐ Require you to "clean your plate" at mealtime
- ☐ Constantly talk about food

The top response to this question was "Require you to 'clean your plate' at mealtime," with 64.2 percent of people choosing that answer. That might have also been the case with you, but listen: You're in a different time and place now. No one is watching over your shoulder and telling you to lick the plate clean. Save the leftovers for another meal, use them for compost, throw them away, whatever works—but please don't use "I was raised this way" as an excuse to con yourself out of reaching your goals. And while we're on the topic—please don't say "I was eating out and I paid for all this so I'm going to eat it," or "It was an all-you-can-eat buffet; I had to stuff myself." I want you to get out of the "clean your plate" mentality and into the "eat until satisfied but not stuffed" frame of mind.

You're setting a new pattern for your mind and body, so your hunger signals will very quickly line up with your new eating routine. You'll likely return to a 3 on the scale after four or so hours have passed following a meal. Anything in between could be mind hunger, or you might be so used to mindless snacking all day that it feels uncomfortable to be at a 4 or 5 on the scale. Again, stick with the new routine and your body will adjust.

You've already taken the important step of removing as many of your external triggers as possible, so you've lowered your risk of eating in reaction to stimuli when you aren't hungry at all. Plus, the foods in this plan were picked because emerging research suggests that they increase satiety (i.e., that feeling of fullness), so you won't find yourself leaving the dinner table unsatisfied and thus rifling through the cupboards for late-night snacks.

Top Seven Tricks for Dealing with Fake Hunger

I want to give you some clear strategies to help overcome mind hunger, because, in my experience, it's often just a matter of getting through the impulse to eat and then you probably won't think about food for a while. Below are some valuable tools for combating that fake, phantom hunger.

First, you've got to understand that if you're entering Phase 1 straight off a 10-day or even a 10-year food bender, where you've been eating anything that crosses your path and you've put nary a thought into the quantities or qualities of the foods you were consuming, then this diet is going to be a shock to your system. Depending on what you've been up to, making a drastic change will likely feel jarring at first. If you've been a chronic muncher, always snacking on something, just the sudden switch to a different eating routine will take some getting used to.

The same goes for your alcohol consumption—if you've been drinking booze every day, you might experience some symptoms of withdrawal when you take that out of the equation. This is all part of reconfiguring your body to switch from "gaining" mode to "losing" mode.

Nobody said this was going to be easy. Remember, this is not one of those diet mirages that falsely promise you an overnight, easy cure for your fat, only to leave you just as heavy as before. This is the real deal, and it's going to take some adjusting. You need to pay close attention to the hunger you're feeling and identify whether it's just your body adapting to your new regimen.

Here are seven tricks you can use to combat fake hunger and cravings. Use them, or let them inspire you to come up with new ones that work for you.

1. Slow down and chew each bite for 30 seconds

Studies indicate that obese people ingest their food quicker and chew their food less than slender people. This is certainly something I have observed with my overweight patients as well. Are you guilty of taking enormous bites, chewing the food barely enough to swallow it, and then immediately going for the next bite? I assure you, there is no reward for eating the fastest or the most food in one sitting.

From now on, I want you to make a conscious effort to slow down, take *much* smaller bites (use a salad fork instead of a dinner fork to make it easier), and spend an entire 30 seconds chewing each bite. Research shows that the extra chewing can actually lower your level of the "hunger hormone," ghrelin, and boost your level of the appetite-suppressing hormone, cholecystokinin. That's right; you can actually create a physiological response in your body that will keep you from overeating, all by slowing down and chewing longer.

2. Turn off the screens

You might think that your smartphone or tablet is your best friend, but did you know it could be causing you to eat more? That's right—a recent study published by the American Academy of Sleep Medicine found that people who were exposed to the type of blue light emitted by this kind of screen before and during an evening meal experienced an acute increase in hunger and insulin resistance. And that's not all; this blue light has also been shown to decrease overall sleepiness, and if you mess with your sleep patterns, you're setting yourself up for even more cases of the munchies the next day.

So, switch off your e-reader or smartphone near mealtime or bedtime. If reading helps you wind down, opt instead for a good, old-fashioned hardcover or paperback book.

3. Revamp your sleep

Catching proper zzz's is a vital aspect to weight loss, especially when you consider one randomized sleep study recently published in the *American Journal of Clinical Nutrition*, which showed that people who sleep less than seven hours per night are predisposed to overeating. In fact, these sleep-deprived study participants consumed an average of nearly 300 calories more per day than those who got enough sleep, and many of those extra calories came from saturated fat. So, make it a priority to get within the ideal range of seven to nine hours of sleep per night.

4. Drink the right stuff

Sometimes when we think we feel hungry, we're actually confusing the signal for thirst with hunger, so it's a smart idea to try drinking a cup of water before reaching for something to eat. Plus, developing research suggests that water may help increase thermogenesis, as scientists observed in one particular study. If you're not a big water drinker, jazz it up with a little squeeze of lemon or go for the sparkling variety.

5. Brush your teeth

Have you ever noticed how bad food tastes if you eat right after you brush your teeth? Use that fact to your advantage and brush your teeth when you're feeling a weak moment coming on.

Because you typically brush your teeth at times of the day when you won't be eating, your brain has an association between minty, fresh breath and non-eating.

6. Call a supporter

Rely on the people to whom you are accountable. Call, text, or e-mail any or all of them for encouragement in the moments that you need it. That's what they're there for!

7. Accomplish a task

You probably know the times of day when you tend to have weak moments—it could be late at night after the kids go to bed, or maybe it's midafternoon or right after work. Prepare for those impulse moments, which most of us experience from four to seven times a day, by having a list of quick tasks you could accomplish instead of giving in and eating. Think about it; there's always a bill to pay, laundry to fold, a car to wash, or an errand to run. Or you could even burn a few extra calories by doing 30 seconds of lunges or jumping jacks. As your concentration shifts to the task at hand, it will move away from thoughts of food. Have some foresight and plan incompatible activities (something you can't do while eating) for those times of day.

When Old Wounds Crowd Out Motivation

Are you struggling with something deeper, an old wound that has played a starring role in your weight problem? Maybe you suffered emotional, physical, or sexual abuse? Were your parents really hard on you growing up? Have you been the victim of ruthless bullying? Perhaps your marriage failed or your spouse cheated?

Whatever the cause of your angst, now is the time to close that book of unfinished emotional business because if you don't, it can stand in the way (once again) of your weight loss success.

I can help you accomplish this through a process I call your Minimal Effective Response (MER). The key word here is "minimal." Now, the *maximum* response might be to shoot the bastard who did this to you, but that has some pretty obvious consequences which lead to a whole new set of problems. Not exactly a winning strategy for healthy closure. But your *minimal* response is something you can do that doesn't cause more trouble and still gives you the maximum result, which is emotional closure.

Here are questions to ask yourself to discover your MER for the situation or person that has caused you harm:

- What action(s) can you take to resolve your emotional pain?

- If you achieve this resolution, how will you feel?

- Does this feeling you will have match the feeling you want to have?

- Knowing we are looking for the minimal response that is still effective for you, is there some other economical action that would give you the resolution you need?

When you do this, you're not saying what happened is acceptable. You're not, in any way, making what they did to you *right*. What you're saying is that you are no longer giving it the ability to crowd out your optimism, your self-esteem, your motivation, or any other positive part of you. You've been tied to this thing for long enough.

All I'm asking you to do is untether, take it off, lay it down, and leave it behind so you can finally say, "OK, I'm done. I'm closing the book on you. This emotional business is finished. Over and out."

Foods That Make You Hungry

As we've been discussing, there are certain foods that research suggests can help you feel full faster and longer, and you're going to be eating a lot of those foods on this plan. But did you know there are foods (probably many of which you eat on a regular basis) that can actually make you feel hungrier and experience *more* cravings? They affect your brain and production of certain hunger hormones so that you constantly want more, more, more—they literally *drive* your hunger. These are very dangerous but also very common foods.

Beware of these potential hunger-inducing food traps:

- Regular and diet sodas
- Concentrated sweeteners including artificial sugars and sugar alcohols (closely check labels for such words as aspartame, sucralose, polydextrose, xylitol, lactitol, mannitol, maltitol syrup, and neotame)
- White bread, pasta, and other starches made with white flour
- Sugary cereals
- Alcohol
- Processed meats (like hot dogs, bacon, and cold cuts)
- Fast food
- French fries and fried chips

You might not have ever realized that these foods can make you feel hungrier and cause you to eat more, but now that you know, you can make a concerted effort to avoid them so they can't derail you. If these are your current everyday staples, don't worry because in the next chapter, you'll learn about the 20/20 Foods that will help you replace your old unhealthy, unhelpful food traps with healthy, helpful alternatives.

In the next chapter, you're going to find out why we chose the 20 foods we did for this diet. These 20/20 Foods are healthy, smart choices for your new way of life to help you reach your weight loss goals.

Coping with Emotional Triggers

I asked about common triggers in our survey. I gave a range of 15 common triggers for overeating or eating unhealthy foods and asked the responders to rate each one on a scale of 1 to 10.

Not surprisingly, 49 percent of people rated "emotions," such as anger, stress, depression, loneliness, or happiness, as their *most* powerful trigger to overeat. The runner-up was "seeking comfort or an escape from physical or emotional pain," which 30.1 percent of respondents rated as their most powerful trigger.

The next time you experience an emotion that typically prompts you to overeat or reach for the bag of chips instead of the apple, follow these steps:

- Take slow, deep breaths in through your nose and exhale out through your mouth for a full 30 seconds.
- Decide how you are going to solve the problem or issue that has arisen. Write down your plan.
- Take action to execute your plan.

Believe it or not, studies have shown that you're actually less able to perceive how much fat is in your food when you are in a heightened state of emotion. This is why it's dangerous to sit down with a tub of ice cream when you're depressed; you're more likely to just eat the whole thing. Now you know what to do instead.

20/20 Instant Intervention: Advertisements for fast food or junk food are targeted not at your hunger pangs but at your innate desire for a better life. They are selling you happiness rather than a bag of French fries. But you've got to beat them at their own game. How do you do that?

The next time you're standing in front of the chips or candy aisle or driving by the fast-food restaurant, think about those commercials that are trying to dupe you, then spend 30 seconds (it will probably take less than 30!) playing the scene all the way to the end. Recall how you felt the last time you ate the junk food.

I mean it—really let yourself experience the fog that came over your brain, the swollen belly, the sluggishness that robbed you of physical activity, and how miserable you felt afterward. As you relive those feelings, push the cart or drive the car away and navigate toward healthy alternatives.

In so doing, you will successfully override the effects that the advertising is meant to have on your brain, and you will have a sense of peace and power because you recognize that you, and only you, are in control of this mission to lose the weight. No matter how many times you gave in and purchased the junk food in your past, today you won.

A massive marketing machine has been jerking you around and programming you to buy their food. You should be mad about that; you have every right to be outraged over their stealthy manipulations. Now that you're alerted to their tactics of selling acceptance rather than food, you can choose not to be played for a fool anymore.

6

STOCK UP ON YOUR 20/20 FOODS

I tried every diet in the book. I tried some that weren't in the book.
I tried eating the book. It tasted better than most of the diets.
—DOLLY PARTON

You're starting to get a handle on right thinking and how to manage and overcome your fake hunger, which is critical. Now let's turn our attention to which foods you should be eating, another crucial component to slimming down once and for all.

There are 20 foods at the core of this diet, and for the first five days, you will be eating only these foods. But don't worry—there are plenty of delicious ways to combine them, and you'll have specific, easy-to-prepare recipes to follow. After those five days, you'll start adding in lots of other tasty and nutritious foods, so don't start panicking that you're going to be confined to just 20 foods for the rest of your life. Remember, I'm not letting you rebel this time, so I'm sticking to my word by making this plan 100 percent doable, even enjoyable.

We've already talked a little about the fact that new theories and emerging research suggest that these foods may be able to assist you in your weight loss goals. Notice I didn't say these foods will miraculously melt all the fat off your hips or thighs if you stuff your face with them 24/7. I am not giving you carte blanche to sit down with a pile of these foods and eat them to your heart's content. You've left that mentality of "eat now, pay later" behind with all the other failed diet gimmicks. Besides, when you listen to your genuine hunger cues, there's no reason to eat nonstop anyway.

What I am saying, however, is that exciting, new research points to certain qualities within these foods that allow them to work with your body to either help you increase thermogenesis, or feel fuller. Unlike those super-restrictive diets that left you hungry enough to eat a box of cookies and the box they came in, I intend to keep you feeling satisfied. Not stuffed, but content and nourished—that's the idea.

The truth is, regardless of their potential to assist you in weight loss, these are healthy, nutritious foods that fuel your body with the right kinds of nutrients. In this list, you won't find any processed, sugar- and salt- or chemical-laden "diet" foods that do you much more harm than good.

They also aren't obscure, exotic, strange foods that you've never heard of (and never cared to); instead, they are everyday superfoods that you can easily (and affordably) get ahold of. They're not your typical "diet" foods either—I haven't just thrown together a food list consisting of the usual suspects of celery and broccoli. These foods taste good, they lend themselves to tons of delicious recipes, and I'm even betting that you already have many of them in your pantry.

High-Response Cost/High-Yield Nutrition

These 20 foods and the meals I'm recommending are all high-response cost/high-yield nutrition foods, a concept you may have first heard me mention in *The Ultimate Weight Solution*. These are foods that take time and effort to prepare and eat. You can't just swallow them whole—they require a little work and chewing. Plus, they provide a lot of nutrition with few calories; in other words, a lot of nutritional bang for your buck.

The balance between fat, fruits, vegetables, protein, and starch that my team and I have created in the meals is ideal for fueling your body with the right nutrients, and you don't have to worry about eating too many calories because the portions are just right. So if you're fretting about how you're going to turn this list into dinner, you can stop stressing because we have done the work for you. You'll learn how to create this balance on your own in the Management Phase too. The recipes throughout the phases of this diet do require a little effort to put together, but we're keeping it simple enough to integrate into your busy life.

Now let's take a look at the theories and new, evolving research that is available for these foods so you can see why we choose them. Again, there's no magic to this. No smoke or mirrors. These are healthy, nutrient-dense foods that fit easily into the low-calorie, sensible meals that we have created. More research is needed to confirm the effects of these foods, but we wanted you to have access to all the latest information to arm you with additional tools to help you reach your goals.

Foods With Potential Thermogenic Properties

New theories suggest that certain foods can boost dietary thermogenesis. Here is some more information about these five foods and how they could help you lose weight:

Coconut oil

The fat in virgin coconut oil is made up of medium-chain triglycerides (MCTs). (Notice I'm talking about virgin coconut oil in its pure form, not coconut oil that has been highly processed or partially hydrogenated.) Scientists believe that MCTs are absorbed quickly and sent directly to the liver, where the body burns them as fuel almost entirely. Some scientists also believe that this process stimulates metabolism and, in some small studies, subjects have experienced an increase in thermogenesis for a short time after ingestion of MCTs compared to LCTs (long-chain triglycerides) alone.

The research on coconut oil is intriguing, but I want you to keep in mind, this is new research that's constantly evolving. Scientists are still not sure what long-term effect MCTs will have on thermogenesis or weight, as not all studies have been positive, but I believe coconut oil can easily be incorporated into a healthy diet, so I thought I wouldn't hold back on giving you this potential tool.

Green tea

You've probably already heard a lot of buzz about green tea and how it promotes weight loss. But, like everything in this diet, you can't just drink a gallon of it or take some green tea extract and expect the weight to fall off of you. (You might have tried that before, and all it did was cause a few extra trips to the bathroom!) Although the jury is still out as to whether green tea leads to weight loss, consuming at least 270 milligrams of epigallocatechin gallate (EGCG) from green tea per day has been shown to increase thermogenesis. We suggest that you aim to drink two to three cups of green tea per day, with at least one of them being caffeinated. Plus you get other great health benefits from drinking green tea.

Mustard

It might be surprising that one of America's favorite condiments could actually offer any benefits other than great taste, but one study involving 25 men published in the *British Journal of Nutrition* suggests that mustard might have the potential to produce diet-induced thermogenesis shortly after consumption compared to the use of other common household spices. More research is needed to confirm the effect and how it can help with weight loss, but mustard is also a low-calorie and delicious way to flavor your foods. So you'll see different types of mustard used in creative ways in several of the recipes within this diet.

Walnuts

Research from one study of 29 men published in the journal *Clinical Nutrition* also suggests that walnuts may have a positive effect on thermogenesis a few hours after consumption as compared to dairy products (which are high in saturated fats). Like the other foods I've described in this section, more research is needed to confirm the effect, but I wanted you to know the latest information and intriguing theories.

Furthermore, walnuts boast high plant-based omega-3 fatty acid content, which is shown to help your body support many basic functions, including digestion, cell growth, and blood clotting.

Olive oil

Researchers also looked at the thermogenic properties of olive oil in the same study I mentioned for walnuts. This emerging research suggests that olive oil, like walnuts, may increase thermogenesis shortly after consumption compared to dairy products. I'm hopeful that more research will be conducted soon to confirm the effects of olive oil.

The nutrition community has been taking a closer look at olive oil in recent years and have been intrigued by its other potential health benefits. For example, some developing research indicates that it may support heart health and cognitive activity. Many dieticians agree that olive oil should be one of the healthy fats included in any well-balanced diet.

Foods That Stick to Your Ribs

The whole point of eating food is to nourish your body when you experience the physical signs of hunger. But, not all foods truly make you feel full and satisfied, and they can fill you up with worthless calories.

However, on the opposite end of that spectrum, there are certain foods that have been shown to make you feel *fuller* and *more* satisfied than other foods in their same category. What follows is some of the new research on them.

Almonds

Almonds, which contain healthy, monounsaturated fats as well as vitamin E and magnesium, have been shown to increase our sense of fullness. A study published in the journal *Nutrition and Metabolism* compared whole almonds to almond butter, almond flour, almond oil, and no almond products to see which had the greatest effect on satiety. Whole almonds showed the strongest results. Almonds have also been shown to support the cardiovascular system and healthy cholesterol.

Apples

These long-extolled, fiber-filled, delicious fruits have been shown to boost the feeling of fullness. Especially when compared to their lesser-celebrated counterparts, apple sauce and apple juice with and without added fiber, whole apples caused subjects to eat less at their next meal, as indicated in a study published in the journal *Appetite*.

Some sayings stand the test of time for a reason, and "an apple a day keeps the doctor away" is one of those. Apples have a chemical called quercetin, which has been shown to support cardiovascular health and immune function.

Chickpeas

Chickpeas, also known as garbanzo beans, are naturally filling due to the high amounts of both protein and fiber found in them. I came across one interesting study published in the journal *Appetite*, and it found that subjects reported a greater perceived satiation (again, feeling of fullness), an improvement in perceived bowel function, and they ate less food in general while consuming chickpeas. One particular finding piqued my interest—it turns out the study participants started eating more processed snack foods once they stopped eating the chickpeas, suggesting that chickpeas might help reduce desire for high-calorie, low-nutrient junk foods. Nutrition experts that I worked with believe that more research is needed to confirm the effects of chickpeas, as not all research has been as positive as this study, but this study is very intriguing and so many tasty dishes can be made with chickpeas. Chickpeas are also high in folate (also commonly known as folic acid), which helps support the health of your heart.

Dried plums (prunes)

You might have an association with prunes that would make you nervous about eating too many of them, but my nutritionist partner, Cynthia, has kept the portions in the recipes just right, so that shouldn't scare you off. A study out of Greece looked at how dried plums affected hunger, and the researchers found that participants who ate snacks that included prunes felt less hungry and had less desire to eat between the snack and their next meal. They concluded that this could be thanks to the high soluble fiber content found in prunes.

It is true that prunes are high in fiber, and they've also been found to have a normalizing effect on blood sugar by slowing down the process of food leaving the stomach. Experts also believe that prunes could support bone health.

Greens (any kind of leafy greens)

Researchers looked at how eating a salad containing iceberg and romaine lettuce before a meal affected fullness and food intake. They found that when study subjects were required to eat a salad before a pasta meal, they tended to eat fewer calories overall and feel fuller. Greens are low in calories, but nutrition experts have theorized they have the ability to produce a feeling of fullness thanks to their volume.

If you haven't heard about the health benefits of leafy greens, then allow me to enlighten you. First of all the choices are vast, so even if you're saying, "I've hated spinach for as long as I can remember," that's OK. I am not telling you to go out and eat a bushel of spinach for dinner. There are many other options that some nutritionists believe will help you feel full, including collard greens, red leaf spinach and lettuce, arugula, and kale. They bring different nutrients and antioxidants to the table (pardon the pun), but they're all great choices for your health and your body. Take a cruise around the produce section of the grocery store and try out a new leafy green you've never had before.

Lentils

The objective of a study conducted at the University of Toronto Department of Nutritional Sciences was to compare how several legumes affect appetite and food intake. They compared chickpeas, lentils, navy beans, and yellow peas to pasta and sauce. They found among other things that a meal with lentils had the strongest impact on satiety, and lentils were the only legume that reduced cumulative food intake, a finding that was compelling to me and my team.

Lentils are a great source of protein, believe it or not, and they also boast a lot of potassium, fiber, iron, B vitamins, magnesium, potassium, and calcium. Yes, they really are that amazing. They're also great either hot (I'm sure you've heard of lentil soup) or cold (you'll see them included in salad recipes later in this book). They're inexpensive nutritional powerhouses.

Peanut butter (natural)

In a study conducted on obese women, Brazilian researchers found that peanut butter, when added to a breakfast meal, helped regulate glucose levels and also increased the production of hormones related to satiety. In other words, it helped the subjects feel full and reduced their desire to eat after the meal.

Peanut butter, when you get an all-natural version that isn't loaded down with sugar, is a healthy source of fat to fuel your body. Look for a peanut butter with no sugar in the ingredients list. It can give you energy, and according to the American Heart Association, the fats in peanut butter don't raise cholesterol.

If you're allergic to peanuts, don't worry. I'll offer you some safe alternatives in Phase 1.

Pistachios (roasted, unsalted)

A study published in the *Journal of the American College of Nutrition* found that of subjects who took part in a weight loss program, the people who ate pistachios as a snack showed a lower body mass index and lower triglycerides when compared to people who ate pretzels as the snack. Despite the fact that pistachios have a relatively high fat content, researchers concluded that pistachios, if portion controlled, may help control body weight. Another study, from the journal *Appetite*, found that when people had to remove the shells from the pistachios versus eating already shelled ones, they actually ate 41 percent fewer without feeling any less satisfied than the other group. So the takeaway message here is to purchase pistachios in their shells so that you have to put in a little extra effort to eat them. The researchers even pointed out that the leftover shells are a good visual reminder of how much you've eaten. And this goes along exactly with what I'm saying about high-response cost foods—you have to work a little to eat them, but it's so worth it.

Pistachios are packed with nutrients such as potassium, magnesium, and vitamin K, as well as some protein and fiber. You've probably heard them referred to as the "skinny nut" because they have the fewest calories of all nuts. But let me caution you again—eating a pound of them a day won't make you skinny.

Raisins

A study published in the journal *Metabolism* found that eating raisins, especially in combination with walking more throughout the day, reduces hunger and helps subjects eat less the rest of the day, possibly because of how they alter hormones related to satiety. Interestingly, they also found that subjects had a decrease in LDL cholesterol as well as reduced post-meal glucose levels.

Raisins also provide your body with a type of antioxidant called anthocyanins, which scientists believe provide many positive health benefits, such as supporting heart health.

Yogurt (nonfat)

When compared to snacks of cheese, milk, and water, yogurt had the greatest ability to suppress appetite, according to a study published in the *British Journal of Nutrition*. The subjects rated their hunger as 24 percent lower after eating yogurt than after eating the cheese or drinking the milk or water. It's important to know—the subjects ate less food later in the day after consuming any of the dairy products in the study, but yogurt did the trick more than the milk or cheese.

Aside from filling you up, yogurt is pretty much a nutritional all-star, as long as you're not eating varieties filled with artificial sweeteners or junky add-ins like chocolate chips. It has healthy bacteria that can support digestion, and it contains calcium. Greek yogurt in particular is typically much higher in protein and lower in sugar overall.

Eggs

There have been several studies regarding how eggs affect fullness, and they all point to the notion that eggs have more of a tendency to "stick to your ribs," especially when compared to carbohydrate-centric meals. Subjects in these studies ate less throughout the day after eating eggs for either breakfast or lunch, and one study even showed that they ate less for the following 36 hours.

There's little doubt that the protein found in eggs is high quality and is often considered to be the standard to which all other forms of protein are compared because of its broad range of amino acids.

Eggs are also good sources of vitamins A, E, and B$_{12}$, and they're inexpensive.

Cod

There have been a few studies looking at how meals consisting of fish protein affect satiety. One study published in the *European Journal of Clinical Nutrition* compared the effects of cod and beef on subjects' hunger and satiety. What they found was that the participants ate less at a meal later that day after having consumed the cod at an earlier meal. What does this mean? Well, it could indicate that cod has the ability to make you feel fuller for longer so that you don't feel the need to eat as much later on.

Codfish is also a low-calorie, delicious type of white fish that is highly versatile in recipes. And with the growing concerns about fish containing dangerous levels of mercury, it's good to know that codfish is among the group of fish with the lowest amount of mercury, according to the Food and Drug Administration. (Other fish typically found to pose a low mercury risk are shellfish, light canned tuna, and smaller ocean fish.) Plus, it's worth mentioning that regularly eating fish can support heart health.

Rye

Whole-grain rye has been shown, in several studies, to increase the feeling of lasting fullness, even when compared to other whole grains such as wheat. Participants in one study published in the journal *Physiology and Behavior* felt a lower desire to eat for the four hours after eating a whole-grain rye breakfast. Some researchers point to the high water-binding capacity of rye fiber (which causes it to stay in your stomach longer) as the possible reason why it increases the sense of fullness.

Whole-grain rye products (such as rye crackers, rye flakes, and rye bread) are healthy complex carbohydrates to include in your diet.

Tofu

Now, I know you might have some trepidation about tofu ("You mean that *mushy* stuff?"), but put your fears aside and give it a try because I think you'll be surprised at just how versatile it is.

Here are just a few reasons why you should learn to love tofu. According to a study published in the journal *Appetite*, when researchers compared the effects of a tofu meal to the effects of a chicken meal, they found that the tofu meal kept the participants full for several hours longer following the meal. Also, soy foods have been found to support healthy blood pressure and cholesterol levels.

Whey protein

Whey protein is one of two major groups of protein found in dairy milk. It's often used in protein shakes and powders. A study published in the *British Journal of Nutrition* compared how meals consisting of whey protein, tuna, turkey, and egg white protein affected participants' satiety. They found that hunger was significantly lower after the whey meal than after the tuna, turkey, and egg meals. The whey protein meal reduced appetite and decreased calorie intake at a later meal compared with the other protein meals, indicating a potential for appetite suppression and weight loss in overweight individuals.

Time-Release Combinations

The new theories and research presented in this section suggest that when you balance carbohydrates, proteins, and healthy fats correctly in your meals, they can create a time-release effect in your body.

My team has used this information to design balanced meals that are meant to make you feel full, and when you reach the Management Phase, you will learn how to create this balance on your own.

Moving into the Three Phases

It's time to move on to the first phase, and as you do, remember: If you frequently choose foods that are nutritionally void, high calorie, or high sugar, you will not get the results you want. Instead, set a new eating pattern for yourself by following the nutritious plan I'm recommending and get ready to watch the number on that scale go down while your energy goes up and you feel much better.

7

PHASE 1:
THE 5-DAY BOOST

Ain't nothin' to it, but to do it.
—Maya Angelou

If you're one of those people whose meals perpetually consist of take-out, delivery, or fast food and you've resorted to using your oven for storing pots and pans, then you need to do a little extra mental preparation before you start this phase. I hope you're sitting down for this piece of news: *healthy eating requires using your kitchen.*

But even if your nightly routine consists of heating up some pack-aged mac 'n' cheese or browning some meat to mix with a box of pasta and sauce, then you might be surprised to learn that these meals are actually *easier* and take the same amount of time as (or less than) those highly processed, unhealthy options you're used to dishing up.

20/20 Instant Intervention: Right now, before you read the recipes for any of these meals, I want you to repeat after me, out loud: "I am not afraid of the kitchen. I promise myself that I will put in the minimal amount of time and effort it takes to prepare these healthy meals, because I owe it to myself to change my relationship with food and food preparation. I don't need to be a gourmet chef in order to feel comfortable in the kitchen and become the master of my kitchen domain, along with the master of my health!"

The 5-Day Boost Guidelines

The first phase is five days long, and your meals will consist exclusively of ingredients from the 20/20 Foods. Like we talked about in the last chapter, new and developing theories and studies suggest that some of these foods may increase thermogenesis, and others help you feel full faster and longer so you're less likely to be hungry later on.

Here is your grocery shopping list for Phase 1:

Foods with Potential Thermogenic Properties

Coconut oil

Green tea

Mustard (yellow or Dijon)

Olive oil

Walnuts

Foods That Stick to Your Ribs

Almonds

Apples

Chickpeas

Dried plums (prunes)

Greens (any kind of leafy greens)

Lentils

Peanut butter (natural)

Pistachios (roasted, unsalted, in
the shell)

Raisins

Yogurt (nonfat)

Eggs

Cod

Rye

Tofu

Whey protein

Four Meals a Day

As I said earlier, each day in this phase you will eat a total of four meals, which are to be spaced about four hours apart from each other. If you're a chronic "muncher," where hardly 10 minutes pass without you chewing on something, this might take a little getting used to. But the reasoning behind this guideline, like every aspect of this diet, is rooted in the latest research.

Allergy Alert

You might have noticed that a few of the foods on the list are commonly associated with allergies, sensitivities, and intolerances. If you know that certain foods on the list cause you problems, you should obviously avoid those. Below are some suggested substitutions, but as with anything related to your physical health, it's best to discuss any new foods with your doctor before introducing them to your diet. If you have an allergy to all tree nuts and you are substituting seeds or seed butters, check the label to make sure they are processed in a facility that does not also process tree nuts. Please note that not all of these foods have been shown in research to have the same effects on thermogenesis or satiety as the foods recommended in the plan.

- Instead of peanut butter, try almonds, hazelnuts, sunflower seeds, or pumpkin butters.
- Instead of walnuts or almonds, try unsalted sunflower seeds or pumpkin seeds.
- For gluten intolerance, gluten allergy, or if you have celiac disease, you can have gluten-free whole-grain bread instead of regular rye bread.
- If you are intolerant or allergic to dairy, including Greek yogurt, you can substitute with a plant-based yogurt or milk, such as almond yogurt or rice milk.
- Instead of whey protein, you can substitute with powders made of brown rice, hemp seed, or pea protein.
- Instead of eggs, you can substitute with another protein source such as tofu or mashed chickpeas.
- If you have an allergy to fish, you can substitute with chicken breast or other lean protein sources.
- Instead of tofu, you can substitute with eggs or a lean protein source such as chicken breast or chickpeas.

For years, the popular thinking has been that eating multiple, small meals throughout the day leads to weight loss. But new theories suggest that eating in this pattern may not actually have any specific weight-related benefits and can, in fact, lead to more hunger. The more you're feeding your body, the more likely you are to be in a constant state of hunger, never feeling fully satisfied, not to mention the fact that the more often you're eating, the more opportunities you have to *over*eat. It can become an ugly cycle.

This plan combats all of that by helping you create a healthy eating pattern with the right foods that satisfy. By the time you're feeling hungry again, it will be time to eat your next meal.

Here are some clear-cut examples of your new meal schedule, but you should really tailor this to your daily routine.

	OR		OR
Breakfast at 6:00 a.m.	Breakfast at 8:00 a.m.		Breakfast at 9:00 a.m.
Snack at 10:00 a.m.	Lunch at 12:00 p.m.		Lunch at 1:00 p.m.
Lunch at 2:00 p.m.	Snack at 4:00 p.m.		Snack at 5:00 p.m.
Dinner at 6:00 p.m.	Dinner at 8:00 p.m.		Dinner at 9:00 p.m.

If none of these realistically apply to you, just stick to the rule of spacing your meals about four hours apart and you'll be on the right track.

Portions for Men

We've done all the work of calculating the portions and proportions for you in Phase 1, but men do need to eat more than women. Guys, your guideline is simple: you should double the portions of ingredients in one meal per day, and that meal needs to be the one right before the most active time of your day. For example, if you work out in the late afternoon, you should double the portions in your lunch or afternoon snack. However, if you work nights or you're on your feet more in the evenings, double the portions in your last meal of the day.

This pattern will work to keep you energized while you're active. You can't "borrow" nutrients from meals you ate hours ago—those

The Truth about Breakfast

You've probably heard that breakfast is the most important meal of the day (maybe you can even hear your own mother's voice reciting it to you), but don't let that be your excuse for waking up to an enormous, sugar-loaded food fest using the faulty rationale that it will keep you from overeating later in the day. A study out of the University of Cambridge found that people who ate a small breakfast in the morning didn't compensate by eating more calories later on. So, it's not the size of the breakfast that matters, just that you start your day with the right kind of fuel to power you through the morning and into the next meal.

are already long gone. That's why you want to plan ahead to double the size of your meals leading up to the time of day when you are the most physically active.

Phase 1 Seasonings

For the first phase, you're going to cleanse your palate and boost your results by using *only* three key seasonings to flavor your foods. Salt is not one of them, and while some sodium in your diet is important, taking a five-day break from adding extra salt to your food will reduce water retention (think: reduction in belly bloat) and teach your taste buds to appreciate the taste of food instead of the taste of salt.

Here are your Phase 1 seasonings:

- Garlic: You've likely heard the buzz about the health benefits of garlic, and the latest theories suggest it could even assist with weight loss.
- Cinnamon: Some studies show that cinnamon could delay emptying of your stomach, so you feel fuller for longer.

- Lemon juice: Packed with high levels of vitamin C, new theories suggest that these yellow wonders may help your body produce an amino acid that could increase thermogenesis.

What to Drink in Phase 1

For the first phase, you should focus on drinking water and green tea. Aim to drink 16 ounces of water with each meal. It's only five days; you can do anything for five days. If you're used to half a bottle of wine every evening with dinner, I know this will be a change. Just remind yourself of your commitment and the real reasons why you're on this weight loss journey.

Let's talk about coffee for a moment, as it's very possible that you are one of the more than 50 percent of Americans over the age of 18 who report drinking coffee at least once a day. Rest easy; you're allowed to have coffee on this plan. Green tea would be a better choice since it's in the list of 20/20 Foods, so if you're able to make the switch, that's great. (Know that green tea contains caffeine, but typically not as much as coffee.) But if I'd have to pry that cup of joe out of your cold, dead hands before you'd let that habit go, it's OK—go ahead and include coffee in Phase 1. Let's be clear: I'm not talking about some high-fat, sugar-saturated whipped dessert masquerading as a coffee. I'm referring to one eight-ounce cup of plain coffee, with no more than a quarter cup of skim or plant-based milk (almond, coconut, rice) and up to one packet or teaspoon of raw sugar (no artificial sweetener). Got that? Pretty simple!

Phase 1 Meals

The idea behind only eating meals using the 20 foods listed above for the first five days is to help you get used to eating the foods in this diet. Here are your Phase 1 meals.

Breakfast Options

APPLE PEANUT BUTTER SMOOTHIE

In blender, combine a single-serve container of nonfat (0%) vanilla Greek yogurt (made with real sugar, not artificial sweetener), a small chopped apple (about 2¾″) of your choice (some options are Red Delicious, Golden Delicious, and Granny Smith) with the skin on, 1/4 cup unsweetened whey protein powder, and 1/4 cup water. Whip until smooth. Add 1 tablespoon natural peanut butter, 1/4 teaspoon cinnamon, and a handful of ice, and whip to desired consistency.

APPLE WALNUT PARFAIT

Chop a small apple (about 2¾″) of your choice (Red Delicious, Golden Delicious, Granny Smith), skin on, and toss with 1/2 tablespoon lemon juice. Layer apple, parfait style, with a single-serve container of nonfat (0%) vanilla Greek yogurt (made with real sugar, not artificial sweetener) and 14 walnut halves, chopped. Sprinkle with cinnamon if desired.

GREEN APPLE SMOOTHIE

In blender, combine a single-serve container of nonfat (0%) vanilla Greek yogurt (made with real sugar, not artificial sweetener), 1 small (about 2¾″) Granny Smith apple, skin on, sliced into chunks, 1/4 cup spinach, 1/4 cup unsweetened whey protein powder, and 2 tablespoons water. Whip until smooth. Add 2 teaspoons coconut oil and a handful of ice and whip to desired consistency.

SPINACH SCRAMBLE

Whisk 1 large egg and season with 1/2 teaspoon minced garlic. In a medium pan, scramble the egg with 1 tablespoon extra-virgin olive oil and 1½ cups fresh spinach. Pair with 1 small (about 2¾″) apple of your choice (Red Delicious, Golden Delicious, Granny Smith), skin on.

BREAKFAST SALAD

Crush or finely chop 1/4 cup shelled pistachios; set aside. In a small bowl, whisk 2 teaspoons Dijon mustard with 1 teaspoon water, 1 teaspoon lemon juice, and 1/4 teaspoon minced garlic. Add 2 cups mixed greens and toss to coat well. Transfer greens to a plate. Sprinkle greens with pistachios and top with 1 large egg, scrambled, sunny-side up, poached, or hard boiled, or 1 serving (1/5 of a 14-ounce package) pan-warmed extra-firm tofu.

Lunch/Dinner Options

APPLE COCONUT SALAD

Crush or finely chop 1/4 cup shelled pistachios; set aside. Chop a small apple (about 2¾″) of your choice (Red Delicious, Golden Delicious, Granny Smith), skin on, and toss with 1/2 tablespoon lemon juice. Sauté in 1/2 tablespoon coconut oil over medium heat until tender. Top 2 cups fresh mixed greens with sautéed apple and sprinkle with pistachios.

DRIED PLUM AND COCONUT SMOOTHIE

In blender, combine a single-serve container of nonfat (0%) vanilla Greek yogurt (made with real sugar, not artificial sweetener), 5 dried plums, 1/4 cup unsweetened whey protein powder, and 1/4 cup water. Whip until smooth. Add 1/2 tablespoon coconut oil, 1/4 teaspoon cinnamon, and a handful of ice, and whip to desired consistency.

EGG SALAD ON RYE CRISP

In a small bowl, whisk 2 teaspoons Dijon mustard with 1 teaspoon water, 1 teaspoon lemon juice, and 1/4 teaspoon minced garlic. Toss with 1 chopped hard-boiled egg. Spoon egg salad over 2 whole-grain rye crackers. Enjoy with 1 small apple (about 2¾″) of your choice (Red Delicious, Golden Delicious, Granny Smith). (Option: replace egg with 1/5 of a 14-ounce package extra-firm tofu, diced.)

Lentil Walnut Salad

Lay 14 walnut halves on a cookie sheet and bake in a preheated 350°F oven for 8 minutes to toast. Chop toasted walnuts and set aside. In a small bowl, whisk 2 teaspoons Dijon mustard with 1 teaspoon water, 1 teaspoon lemon juice, and 1/4 teaspoon minced garlic. Add 1/2 cup cooked lentils (boiled, steamed, or canned; drained and rinsed) and toss to coat. Spoon lentils over 2 cups fresh mixed greens and sprinkle with walnuts. (Option: leave walnuts raw.)

Greens Over Almond Cod

Chop 1/4 cup whole unsalted raw or dry-roasted almonds; set aside. In a shallow dish, bake 4 ounces of fresh cod fillet at 350°F for 10 minutes, or until fish easily flakes with fork. Sauté 2 cups mixed greens in 1 teaspoon extra-virgin olive oil and 1/4 teaspoon minced garlic. Place cod fillet on plate, cover with sautéed greens, garnish with chopped almonds, and serve with fresh lemon.

Chilled Cod Salad

Crush or finely chop 2 tablespoons unsalted raw or dry-roasted almonds; set aside. In a small bowl, whisk 2 teaspoons Dijon mustard with 1 teaspoon water, 1 teaspoon lemon juice, and 1/4 teaspoon minced garlic. Toss with 3 ounces cooked, chilled, flaked cod fillet, 1 cup finely chopped spinach, and the chopped almonds. Spoon onto 2 rye crisps.

Cod Cakes

In a medium bowl, lightly mash 1/2 cup chilled lentils (boiled, steamed, or canned; drained and rinsed). Add 1/4 cup chopped spinach, 2 teaspoons Dijon mustard, 1 teaspoon water, 1 teaspoon lemon juice, and 1/4 teaspoon minced garlic. Fold in 3 ounces cooked, flaked cod fillet and 2 crushed rye crisps. Form into three round cod cakes and bake on a cookie sheet (lightly misted with olive oil nonstick spray) in a preheated 350°F oven for 5 minutes on each side.

PB&P

Spread 1 tablespoon all-natural peanut butter on 2 whole-grain rye crackers. Sprinkle with cinnamon if desired and enjoy with 5 dried plums. (Option: slice dried plums and place on top of peanut butter.)

ROASTED CHICKPEA PICNIC

Preheat oven to 350°F. Toss 1/2 cup chickpeas (boiled or canned; rinsed and drained) with 2 teaspoons extra-virgin olive oil and 1/4 teaspoon minced garlic. Spread out on cookie sheet and roast for 10 minutes. Serve with a small apple of your choice (Red Delicious, Golden Delicious, Granny Smith) and 2 whole-grain rye crackers. (Option: chickpeas can be roasted ahead of time, stocked in fridge, and enjoyed chilled.)

SPINACH HUMMUS

In a blender or food processor, purée 1/2 cup chickpeas, 2 teaspoons extra-virgin olive oil, 1/2 teaspoon minced garlic, 1 tablespoon lemon juice, 2 tablespoons water, and 1/2 cup fresh spinach (add more water, 1 tablespoon at a time, if needed). Serve hummus with wedges of a small apple of your choice (Red Delicious, Golden Delicious, Granny Smith), skin on.

EASY BREEZY RAISINS AND ALMONDS

Enjoy 1/4 cup each raisins and unsalted raw or dry-roasted almonds.

SONOMA TOFU SALAD

Chop 1 tablespoon raw or dry-roasted unsalted walnuts; set aside. In a small bowl, whisk 2 teaspoons Dijon mustard with 1 teaspoon water, 1 teaspoon lemon juice, 2 teaspoons olive oil, and 1/4 teaspoon minced garlic. Add crumbled tofu (1/5 of a 14-ounce package extra-firm tofu), 1 tablespoon raisins, and the chopped walnuts. Serve with 2 rye crisps.

Meals with Meaning

In chapter 3, I asked you to write down everything you ate for one full day and what you were thinking about when you ate it. Most of the time, people tell me they had absolutely no clue how much they were really eating on a daily basis. Right now, I want you to go back and look at what you were thinking about when you ate those foods.

Were you thinking about how stressed out you were? Or how lonely you felt? Or maybe you were thinking about how much fun you were having while taking down whole trays of finger foods at a party. Were you eating out of habit—your regular 3:00 p.m. snack off the dollar menu? Or perhaps were you totally devoid of thought and as soon as you wolfed down the food, you seemed to instantly forget it. Well, my aim is to get you out of these mindsets and into one of assigning value to the food you are eating.

Before you begin eating each meal, I want you to perform a 30-second pre-meal check-in. Use this time to remind yourself of your goal weight and the core reasons why you're choosing to eat healthier and lose weight. Or, think about how this meal will fuel your body so you can accomplish more, have more energy to spend time with your family, think more clearly at work, and so on.

Whatever you do, try to assign positive meaning to the food you are about to eat so you can begin to think of these foods as giving you a physical and mental *reward*. Each time you put a morsel of food in your mouth is an opportunity to think about the meaning behind what you're doing—returning to health and achieving your get-real weight, because you now have a personal truth that requires it of you.

In addition to a 30-second pre-meal check-in with yourself, here are techniques I first introduced in *The Ultimate Weight Solution* for eating less at each sitting. In fact, I bet you'll enjoy each meal more because you'll be eating mindfully.

- When you sit down to a meal, wait five minutes to start eating.

- Put your fork down between bites; finish swallowing before your next bite.

- Eat slowly, and take a break halfway through the meal so your brain can register what you've eaten.

- Do not eat while on the move; sit down at the table.

- Eliminate distractions that cause mindless eating, such as the TV, computer, or phone.

- Leave some food on your plate; you can always save it for later.

Where Does Exercise Fit In?

In chapter 10, you will find out about the 30-Second Burn Burst Exercise Program. I think you will find it to be highly effective and easy to integrate into your lifestyle. I encourage you to check out that chapter before you begin Phase 1.

Moving on to Phase 2: The 5-Day Sustain

The first phase is only five days long, and the same goes for the next phase. Once you've completed the three phases, you might return to Phase 1 if you have more weight to lose; it's a great and healthy way to jump-start your results.

8

PHASE 2:
THE 5-DAY SUSTAIN

The three great essentials to achieve anything worthwhile are, first,
hard work; second, stick-to-itiveness; third, common sense.
—THOMAS A. EDISON

After you've completed the 5-Day Boost, it's critical that you take a moment to reflect on how you're feeling and to take notice of the changes occurring in your body and your mind. Right now, flip back to chapter 4 and write down your weight and measurements now that you've completed Phase 1. It's also imperative to note the other changes you're experiencing. They might be subtle or they might be quite obvious. Use the questions below to guide your assessment.

Acknowledging Your Progress

Do you notice an improvement in your energy level
throughout the day?   Yes   No

Do you feel more mentally focused and alert?   Yes   No

Do you notice any improvement in your respiration?
For example, are you breathing easier during exercise
than when you first started?   Yes   No

Have you noticed a reduction in your hunger and
cravings?   Yes   No

Are you feeling healthier overall? In other words, have you noticed an intangible feeling that you might now live longer and feel better about yourself and your choices?   Yes No

Has your digestion improved? For example, are you noticing less heartburn, belly bloating, trouble with bowel movements, stomachaches, etc.?   Yes No

Do you feel more in control of your eating and exercise habits?   Yes No

Any progress is good progress, so write down anything else positive you might be feeling and experiencing.

....

....

....

....

....

Celebrate your improvements and each incremental goal as you reach it—just not with food of course.

Set Up Your Healthy Reward System

Pop quiz: How have you rewarded yourself when you've lost weight in the past? I ask because it's important to celebrate your achievements every step of the way, but let's talk about exactly how you've been rewarding yourself. For instance, have you ever found yourself jumping off the scale, thrilled with your new weight, and then racing to the nearest form of junk food because you've "earned a reward"? You might think, "I'm down 10 pounds! I have got to get me a few slices of pizza!"

How ludicrous is that? Now that you're losing weight in the right way, I don't want you to jeopardize it by "rewarding" yourself with what really amounts to a punishment. Instead, you've got to set up a healthy reward system. The truth is, if you can just manage to get through that one, impulsive moment of weakness, you will be all set for hours. It won't keep returning to nudge you toward the plate of brownies (which I hope isn't even *in* your new, no-fail household, by the way!). You'll get over the hump and then it will be smooth sailing until your next meal.

Some examples of sensible rewards that are not food related include having a massage, facial, manicure, or pedicure; taking a bubble bath while reading a book; or playing outside with the kids or pets.

You could also set up incentives for each weight loss milestone you reach. One study shows that people who have cash incentives to lose weight actually tend to lose more. So maybe you start a pool or friendly competition with friends.

Write your list of rewards and keep it near you so that when you feel like "rewarding" yourself in a negative way, you have healthy options right at your fingertips.

My Healthy Reward List

....

....

....

....

....

The 5-Day Sustain Guidelines

Now that you are ready for the second phase, which is also only five days long, you'll start enjoying more foods in addition to the 20/20 Foods. Just like Phase 1, you'll have a list of nutritionally balanced meals that we've created for you, and you'll notice that each meal includes at least two of the 20/20 Foods as well as a protein source. You'll continue to space out your four daily meals by approximately four hours.

Because we want to avoid rebellion, we're switching things up a little in Phase 2 by adding more variety. These new foods will also offer a whole host of nutritional benefits, and give you the range of vitamins and minerals your body needs.

Here they are:

Power Proteins	Super Starches
Chicken breast	Oats
Tuna (chunk light, canned in water)	Brown rice
	Corn
Black beans	

Prime Produce—Veggies	Fit Fats
Carrots	Avocado
Tomatoes	Sunflower seeds
Mushrooms	Cashews

Prime Produce—Fruits

Blueberries

Oranges

Grapes

Why Are These Foods Added in Phase 2?

We picked this specific list of foods to add into the second phase for several reasons. The "power proteins" listed here offer a high protein content, with low saturated fat. They are all lean proteins, which according to emerging research, can help increase thermogenesis and help maintain muscle. They also bring other essential and energy-providing vitamins and nutrients to the mix. These foods are easy to find at any grocery store, they're inexpensive, and they're delicious.

The "prime produce" fruits and vegetables made the list because they are rich in vibrant colors, and those colors are tied to health-protecting antioxidants. For example, tomatoes get their red color from pigments called lycopene, and carrots get their orange hue from beta-carotene. These tasty vegetables act as powerful antioxidants in our bodies. Needless to say, fresh fruits and vegetables are also rich in essential vitamins.

The "super starches" are standouts because they are whole grains, which means they are sources of complex carbohydrates that your body needs. In their whole, unprocessed forms (meaning their bran and germ haven't been removed), these starches are delicious and filling additions to your balanced meals. You need super starches because of their B vitamins and key minerals; plus, they provide slow-burning energy. Carbohydrates are your body's preferred fuel source, but the portions in these meals are designed to fuel your daily activity without creating surpluses that prevent you from losing fat.

The "fit fats" added in this second phase offer your body heart-healthy fats. These foods are also packed with vitamins, minerals, and fiber, all of which play key roles in accomplishing the goals of this phase. They also increase your body's satiety, so you feel fully satisfied for longer periods of time, and they increase your body's absorption of antioxidants and vitamins.

These categories by themselves are important, but as we talked about earlier, the way they're combined within each meal is also significant. The combination of antioxidant-rich produce, wholesome starch, lean protein, and heart-healthy fat provides a broad spectrum of nutrients at every meal. They also complement each other in important ways. For example, the protein works together with the starches by slowing down your digestion of healthy starches; this better regulates your blood sugar and insulin levels and thus provides your body with carbohydrate fuel in a time-released manner. The result is better blood sugar and insulin regulation. (In other words, no sugar highs and crashes.) Likewise, fats work well with proteins to provide the raw materials your body needs for healing and repairing cells. The idea is to eat these foods together at each meal to maximize their benefits. It's not just what you eat; your meals also have to have the proper balance. With the meal options you'll find later in this chapter, I've taken out all the guesswork for you.

Practice Sensible Splurging

Perfectly adhering to any diet 100 percent of the time is a challenge in the real world, and that's where both you and I live. By starting this diet, you are not entering into some kind of parallel universe where you suddenly don't want to eat anything except the foods listed here. But I don't want you to experience the guilt commonly associated with "cheating" on a diet. Instead, I want you to get into the mindset of "sensible splurging." Here's how it works.

Starting in Phase 2, you are allowed a sensible splurge once or twice a week. Studies show that people who know there is a splurge available to them tend to actually splurge less and be more successful on weight loss programs. Just knowing that you *can* have a splurge is often enough to satisfy you, and you don't have to actually follow through with it. Sure, you might be thinking, "Oh great, this is some psychobabble that's just trying to talk me out of my glass of wine." No, it's really not, because I'm also telling you that you can absolutely have the splurge and it will not totally derail your weight loss, if you follow the rules. That's a big "if" there, and I want to make sure you caught it. There are rules for this—having a splurge does not mean going rogue.

First, you need to understand what a sensible splurge looks like. Because if you think a bucket of popcorn the size of your head or a king-size candy bar you picked up in the checkout line is "sensible," you are kidding yourself. A reasonable splurge portion should not exceed approximately 100 calories. Here are some examples:

4-ounce glass of red or white wine

14 potato chips

2 store-bought chocolate chip cookies

1-ounce bar of dark chocolate

4 oz. gummy bears

2 bite-size candy bars

3 vanilla wafer cookies

Before you indulge in a splurge, I want you to complete a 30-second assessment. Here are the questions:

- Is there an emotional reason why I want this splurge (sadness, stress, or boredom) and if so, is there another way I can address the emotion without turning to food?
- Is it enough just knowing that a splurge is allowed and available to me, so I can skip it this time?
- Would a glass of regular or sparkling water or a cup of tea help this desire pass?
- Can I distract myself from this desire for a splurge by doing another activity (take a bath, go on a short walk, etc.)?

Make an honest effort to bypass the splurge if you can. Even doing so occasionally will demonstrate to you that it's actually not that bad to go without it. If, however, the answer to all four of the above questions is "no," then go ahead with the splurge, but ONLY if you have already exercised or will definitely be exercising later that day. That exercise is a key component to making these splurges fit into your overall weight loss plan.

If you're worried about not being able to stop at a 100-calorie splurge, remember that, beyond that amount, it will start to harm your efforts to reach your goals. You have now attached consequences, either positive or negative, to your behavior so you'll find that you're able to control it better than ever.

Phase 2 Seasonings

In Phase 1, you seasoned your meals exclusively with garlic, cinnamon, or lemon. The idea was to let your body and taste buds get used to enjoying the taste of healthy foods while you rid yourself of excess sodium and help reduce your cravings for salt. The goal is to get you to a point where you don't even miss the salt, and if you were to take a bite of one of the salt-laden foods that you used to eat on a daily basis, you'd probably want to spit it out immediately. The same goes for sugar—I want you to feel like even your formerly favorite sweets are overpowering because you are now conditioned differently.

In the second phase, you can start adding in some additional seasonings to your meal routine if you want to. Select salt-free seasonings (such as fresh or dried herbs) that produce a flavor and aroma that satisfies your hankerings. As you'll see, we've already added new seasonings to the meals in this phase, including cilantro, crushed red pepper, and Italian herbs, but it's perfectly OK to add more variety if you'd like.

Phase 2 Meals

When it comes to portion sizes, it's important that you continue to learn by doing, which means sticking to the portions and proportions we've designed for you in these meals. The ingredients work together to give your body the right balance of protein, fat, fiber, and carbohydrates so that you are energized and satisfied but not stuffed.

The same rule applies for men as in Phase 1: double the portion of one meal each day, before your most active time of day.

Breakfast Options

BLUEBERRY ALMOND OATMEAL

Chop 2 tablespoons unsalted raw or dry-roasted almonds; set aside. In a small bowl, mix together 1/4 cup each unsweetened whey protein powder and rolled oats. Prepare with hot water to desired consistency (suggested 1/4 cup) and add a dash of cinnamon. Top with 1 cup fresh blueberries and the chopped almonds. (Options: use 3/4 cup frozen, thawed blueberries in place of fresh; use sliced almonds.)

Mexi Omelet

Whisk 1 large egg and season with 1/4 teaspoon minced garlic and 1 tablespoon chopped cilantro (optional). In a medium pan, cook the egg with 1 cup fresh spinach and 1/2 cup frozen, thawed corn. Top with 1/4 of a ripe avocado, sliced. Pair with 1 small (about 2¾″) apple of your choice (Red Delicious, Golden Delicious, Granny Smith), skin on.

Orange Parfait

Layer a single-serve container of nonfat (0%) vanilla Greek yogurt (made with real sugar, not artificial sweetener) with chopped sections from 1 small orange (seeds removed), 2 tablespoons rye flakes, and 2 tablespoons raw or dry-roasted, unsalted sunflower seeds. (Option: replace rye flakes with rolled oats and pair parfait with green tea so you still have two 20/20 Foods.)

Peanut Butter Raisin Spread

Place 2 tablespoons natural peanut butter in a small bowl. Warm in the microwave for 30–45 seconds. Immediately stir in 1½ tablespoons unsweetened whey protein powder, 1 tablespoon water, and 1 tablespoon each raisins and dry rolled oats. Serve as a spread with 1 small (about 2¾″) apple of your choice (Red Delicious, Golden Delicious, Granny Smith), skin on, sliced.

Green Grape Smoothie

In blender, combine a single-serve container of nonfat (0%) vanilla Greek yogurt (made with real sugar, not artificial sweetener), 3/4 cup green grapes, 1/4 cup spinach, 1/4 cup unsweetened whey protein powder, and 2 tablespoons water. Whip until smooth. Add 1/4 of a ripe avocado, 1 tablespoon rye flakes, and a handful of ice and whip to desired consistency.

CHILLED CHICKEN CORN SALAD

In a medium bowl, combine 1 tablespoon extra-virgin olive oil, 1/2 tablespoon balsamic vinegar, 1/2 teaspoon minced garlic, 1 tablespoon chopped cilantro (optional), 3 ounces diced cooked boneless, skinless chicken breast, and 1/2 cup frozen, thawed corn. Serve over 1 cup of greens of your choice, or toss with the greens.

TUNA SALAD OVER GREENS

Chop 2 tablespoons walnuts; set aside. In a small bowl, combine 3 ounces chunk light tuna canned in water (drained, rinsed) with 1½ tablespoons balsamic vinegar, 1/4 teaspoon salt-free dried Italian herb seasonings, and 1/2 cup cooked and chilled brown rice. Serve over 1 cup greens of your choice (baby spinach, arugula, watercress, romaine) and garnish with the walnuts.

OPEN-FACED EGG AVOCADO SALAD SANDWICH

In a small bowl, combine 1/4 of a ripe avocado, mashed, with 1/4 teaspoon minced garlic, 1/8 teaspoon crushed red pepper (optional), and 1 large chopped hard-boiled egg. Spoon onto 1 slice (1 ounce) whole-grain rye bread and serve with 1 cup baby carrots and 1/4 cup fresh seedless grapes. (Option: if you can't find 100 percent whole-grain rye bread, look for a multigrain 100 percent whole-grain bread that includes rye, or use a different 100 percent whole-grain bread and pair with green tea.)

CHICKEN AVOCADO LETTUCE WRAPS

In a small bowl, combine 1/4 of a ripe avocado, mashed, with 1/4 teaspoon minced garlic, 1/8 teaspoon black pepper, and 3 ounces diced cooked boneless, skinless chicken breast. Fill 2 outer romaine lettuce leaves with mixture and top with 2 crushed rye crisps.

Black Bean and Veggie Platter

In a medium pan, sauté 1 cup spinach, 1/2 cup chopped mushrooms, and 1/4 cup sliced grape tomatoes in 1 tablespoon extra-virgin olive oil, 1/4 cup low-sodium vegetable broth, 1/2 teaspoon minced garlic, and a pinch of cayenne pepper (optional). When mushrooms are tender, add 1/2 cup cooked black beans (boiled or low-sodium canned) and heat through. Serve over 1/2 cup cooked brown rice (fluffy, not packed).

Snack Options

Apple Cashew Muesli

Chop 2 tablespoons cashews (raw or unsalted, dry roasted); set aside. In a small bowl, combine a single-serve container of nonfat (0%) vanilla Greek yogurt (made with real sugar, not artificial sweetener) with 1 small (about 2¾″) apple of your choice (Red Delicious, Golden Delicious, Granny Smith), skin on, sliced, 1 tablespoon rolled oats, 1/8 teaspoon ground cinnamon, and cashews. Chill in refrigerator at least 30 minutes.

Peppery Avocado Chickpea Crackers

In a small bowl, combine 1/4 of a ripe avocado, mashed, with 2 teaspoons lemon juice, 1/2 teaspoon minced garlic, a pinch of black pepper, and 1/8 teaspoon crushed red pepper. Fold in 1/2 cup chickpeas (boiled or canned; rinsed and drained) to coat. Spoon mixture on top of 2 whole-grain rye crisps and serve with 1/2 cup each grape tomatoes and baby carrots.

Grab-'n'-Go Sunny Snack

Enjoy 1 medium orange, a large hard-boiled egg, 2 whole-grain rye crisps, and 2 tablespoons raw or roasted sunflower seeds. (Option: slice egg and place on top of crackers.)

Blueberry Peanut Butter Smoothie

In blender, combine a single-serve container of nonfat (0%) vanilla Greek yogurt (made with real sugar, not artificial sweetener), 3/4 cup frozen unsweetened blueberries, 1/4 cup unsweetened whey protein powder, and 1/4 cup water. Whip until smooth. Add 1 tablespoon each natural peanut butter and rolled oats along with a handful of ice and whip to desired consistency.

Hummus and Crunchy Carrots

In a blender or food processor, purée 1/2 cup chickpeas, 2 teaspoons extra-virgin olive oil, 1/2 teaspoon minced garlic, and 1 tablespoon lemon juice. Serve hummus with 1 cup raw baby carrots and 2 rye crisps.

Dinner Options

Chicken with Garlic Dill Corn and Veggie Sauté

Bake or grill 3 ounces boneless, skinless chicken breast. Sauté 2 cups fresh spinach and 1/2 cup frozen, thawed corn in 1 tablespoon extra-virgin olive oil with 1/2 teaspoon minced garlic and 1 teaspoon fresh or 1/2 teaspoon dried dill. Spoon corn and veggie sauté over chicken.

Lemon Pepper Chicken Pasta

In a medium pan, sauté 1/2 cup sliced grape tomatoes in 1 tablespoon extra-virgin olive oil with 1/2 teaspoon minced garlic until tomatoes are slightly tender. Toss sautéed tomatoes with 1/2 cup cooked whole-grain rye pasta, 1 cup fresh spinach, 1/2 tablespoon lemon juice, 1/4 teaspoon black pepper, and 3 ounces diced cooked boneless, skinless chicken breast.

Lentil Sauté

In a medium saucepan, sauté 1 small plum tomato, minced, and 1 cup greens of your choice (baby spinach, arugula, watercress, romaine) in 2 tablespoons low-sodium vegetable broth, 2 teaspoons extra-virgin olive oil, with 1/2 teaspoon minced garlic and 1/4 teaspoon salt-free dried Italian herb seasonings. Add 1/2 cup cooked lentils (boiled, steamed, vacuum sealed, or canned; drained and rinsed) and heat through. Serve over 1/2 cup cooked brown rice (fluffy, not packed).

Mushroom Tofu Stir-Fry

In a medium pan, stir together 1 tablespoon coconut oil, 1/2 teaspoon minced garlic, 1/4 cup low-sodium vegetable broth, and 1/8 teaspoon crushed red pepper. Add 1/2 cup greens of your choice (spinach, Chinese spinach, kale, chard) and 1 cup sliced mushrooms and sauté until mushrooms are slightly tender. Add cubed extra-firm tofu (1/5 of a 14-ounce package) and heat through. Place sautéed veggies and tofu over a bed of 1/2 cup cooked brown rice (fluffy, not packed).

Walnut Cod with Roasted Carrots

Slice 2 large carrots into thin bite-size chunks at a 45-degree angle, chop or crush 2 tablespoons walnuts; set both aside. Place 4 ounces fresh cod in a shallow pan and sliced carrots on a cookie sheet. Place both in preheated 350°F oven and check often after 6 minutes. Remove cod when fish easily flakes with a fork and carrots when tender. Place cod on a bed of 1/2 cup cooked brown rice (fluffy, not packed), garnish with walnuts, and serve with carrots, along with wedges of fresh lemon.

As you begin to lose weight, I want you to be on your guard against potential saboteurs and decide how you will deal with them. These are the people in your life who are likely to encourage you to "cheat" because they are insanely jealous when others start to lose weight or better themselves in any way. They want to see you go down, and I'm not talking about the number on the scale.

You know what I'm talking about here. We asked our national sample whether they had ever felt sabotaged or resented by a friend, spouse, or family member when they were losing weight. The results: 41.6 percent of you answered "yes."

We as humans can be very petty. If you go out to dinner with a bunch of your overweight friends and you've lost 40 pounds, you are very threatening to them. They'll say, "Come on, don't be a stick-in-the-mud. You're no fun anymore." But you know better. That's got jealousy written all over it.

Sometimes a saboteur comes in the form of a well-intentioned family member who shows their love for you with food. I come from the South, so I know all about this. We'd go for a visit and my family would be slaughtering hogs, killing chickens, frying up pounds of potatoes, gravy, pies, all of it—that was my mother's way of loving us. Whether it's well-meaning or not, you have to be willing to look these folks in the eye and say something like this:

"I'm having a great time and I'm really excited for us to all be together. I'm working hard to improve my health, lose weight, and adjust my lifestyle, and kind of like an alcoholic, I really don't want to fall off the wagon. Thank you so much for understanding and supporting me in what I'm doing."

Depending on the type of saboteur you're dealing with, your response might differ. But what you can do right now is anticipate the sabotage, prepare yourself for it and put your guard up against it so it can't throw you off the course when it does actually occur.

You need to have some pat responses, like the script I just gave you, at the ready. Doing this exercise will help you steel yourself against any potential threats to your success.

A word of caution: As your excitement about losing weight builds, make sure you don't let your gung-ho attitude cross over into "self-righteous know-it-all" territory. If you find yourself telling everybody else what they should or shouldn't be eating and preaching your new knowledge about healthy foods, it's time to put a cork in it. They don't want you spewing your new wisdom all over them—it can come off as very obnoxious. A definite turnoff.

Make Your Social Media Accounts Work for You

If you use them appropriately, your social media accounts can actually help instead of hinder your weight loss efforts. One study out of the University of South Carolina showed that people who posted information about their weight loss as they dieted lost more weight. It's all in how you set up your virtual environment.

If you get involved in online weight loss support groups, post photos of your healthy food choices as a visual food journal, or just celebrate your success with like-minded friends online, this experience can enhance your weight loss.

Moving toward Phase 3: The 20-Day Attain

After you've completed the second phase, you should be feeling much more in control of your behavior and your diet. You are 10 days into the diet, and you're settling into a new pattern, which is very motivating. Now that you have completed the necessary preparation work—physically, psychologically, and beyond—you are ready for the next 20 days, which are the heart of the 20/20 Diet. You've looked backward, you've looked forward, and you've got all the vision you need to make your get-real weight a reality.

9

PHASE 3:
THE 20-DAY ATTAIN

Success is not final, failure is not fatal: it is the courage to continue that counts.
—Sir Winston Churchill

You've now been following this plan for 10 days—congratulations! The past 10 days have essentially been preparation for the 20-Day Attain phase, which is truly the crux of this diet. You have laid the important groundwork, and you're likely feeling better than you have in a long time.

Let's perform another quick self-evaluation so you can really see and appreciate your progress. Go back to chapter 4 and fill in your updated weight and measurements, then answer the questions below. Remember to reward yourself in a healthy way for your achievements.

Acknowledging Your Progress

Have you continued to feel improvement in your energy
levels throughout the day?   Yes   No

Do you continue to feel more mentally focused and alert?   Yes   No

Is exercise becoming easier for you to complete?   Yes   No

Are you more aware of your physical hunger and are you
handling cravings with more ease?   Yes   No

Are you feeling healthier and lighter overall?   Yes   No

Do you feel more in control of your eating and exercise
habits?   Yes   No

Write down anything else positive you might be feeling and
experiencing.

....

....

....

....

In the third phase, which is 20 days in length, you'll be adding in
a wide variety of food to keep your palate from getting bored, to stop
any hint of rebellion you might experience, and to give your body the
essential nutrients it needs. (So if you've been missing a particular fruit
or vegetable, you'll probably find it in this phase.) Each meal will still
include at least two of the 20/20 Foods, and you'll even have some
recommendations for how and what to order out at restaurants. For
you to get what you want out of this journey and to maintain your
positive results, you need a solid plan in place for all circumstances,
and that certainly includes eating out.

The 20-Day Attain Guidelines

To keep you on track with the nutritional content and balance of your
meals, there are still specific recipes from which you'll choose all your
meals in Phase 3.

Variety is a key component to weight loss success, so there are 80
meals (in appendix B) that you can rotate in any way you like for the
next 20 days. You might find specific ones that you love and want to
repeat over and over, which is perfectly fine. Or you might want to
try each of them once! Either way, I encourage you to have fun with
these, and start to make this new healthy way of eating your permanent lifestyle.

This isn't about becoming a gourmet chef and spending hours preparing meals every day. That's not realistic for most of us. And that's

also why these meals don't require culinary training or lots of free time; they are quick, easy, and designed for people with little or no cooking experience.

This phase contains some important carryovers from the previous phases:

Consistent Meal Spacing: By now, you've likely acclimated to eating approximately every four hours. In this phase, continue with the routine of consuming four meals per day, every four hours. This consistent meal schedule is a healthy, efficient way for your body to function. By the time you're hungry, we're feeding you again, which not only keeps you from rebelling, but it helps you burn more calories continuously throughout the day.

Keep using the 20/20 Hunger and Fullness Scale in chapter 5 so you can decipher physical hunger from fake, trigger-induced, or habit hunger and so you don't overeat at mealtime. If you're full, stop eating! You should be letting go of that desire to lick your plate clean.

Splurge Sensibly: As you did in Phase 2, follow the rules for sensible splurging, knowing that you are capable of having a handful of something once or twice a week, but just don't turn it into a pig-out session. You can accomplish your goals without feeling like you'll never be able to enjoy another piece of chocolate or glass of wine.

Eat Out Responsibly: Speaking of restriction, you shouldn't have to swear off restaurants for the remainder of your life in order to succeed at weight loss. But you do need to be armed with a clear-cut game plan before you place your order. Let's spend some time talking about strategies for eating out.

Guidelines for Eating Out

When you go out to a restaurant, you're entering back into an environment in which you will be surrounded by the sights, smells, and sounds associated with triggers and temptations. The only way to keep yourself on track and out of trouble is to know exactly what you're going to order before you even get in the car. This kind of active foresight takes barely any time at all, and the payoff is big. Spend just a few seconds deciding what you're going to eat and drink before you go and you'll guarantee that you will leave that restaurant feeling satisfied (not stuffed) and beaming with pride that you got through the trigger gauntlet without one slipup.

Many restaurants now offer online menus, so you can review your options ahead of time. If not, don't worry. Given the variety of food available to you in Phase 3, you can bank on the fact that most restaurants offer some basics that will work great for you.

Restaurant Rules

1. As with all your meals, make sure this one includes at least two of the 20/20 Foods.

2. Green tea could be one of those options, and it's widely available.

3. If you're comfortable with it, you could bring one of the foods with you to the restaurant (such as almonds, rye crisps, raisins—all very portable).

4. If you're uncomfortable bringing your own ingredient(s), you could eat one of them right before you go to the restaurant.

5. Make sure the restaurant meal contains:
   - Prime produce (fruit and/or veggies)
   - Power protein
   - Super starch (a 100 percent whole-grain item, corn, or skin-on whole potatoes)
   - Fit fat

Restaurant Meal Examples

Here are some sample meals you can order at popular restaurants, and they all follow the above Phase 3 meal requirements. (* indicates bring your own)

BJ's Restaurant and Brewhouse

EnLIGHTened Thai Chicken Mango Salad, add corn and substitute almonds for wonton crisps.

California Pizza Kitchen

Half a Roasted Veggie Salad with grilled shrimp, paired with hot or iced unsweetened green tea*. Order the dressing on the side and use half, or skip the dressing and ask for vinegar to season your salad.

Cheesecake Factory

Seared Tuna Tataki Salad, dress salad with vinegar, fresh-squeezed lemon, and black pepper instead of the wasabi vinaigrette. Add almonds for a 20/20 Food. Make sure to snack on 2 rye crisps before or after your meal to incorporate a "super starch"!

Veggie Burger (no bun) served with mixed greens dressed with oil and vinegar, fresh-squeezed lemon, and black pepper. Ask to substitute mustard for the mayo.

Chili's

Mango-Chile Chicken with corn on the cob (plain, without butter or seasoning) and side salad dressed with vinegar, fresh-squeezed lemon, and black pepper. Pair with green tea*.

Caribbean Salad, add avocado and dress with vinegar, fresh-squeezed lemon, and black pepper and add 1 crumbled rye crisp* for crunch.

Chipotle Mexican Grill

Salad à la carte made with greens, black beans, tomato salsa, corn salsa, and guacamole, paired with hot or iced unsweetened green tea*.

El Pollo Loco

Fire-Grilled Skinless Chicken Breast served with side salad dressed with oil and vinegar, fresh-squeezed lemon, and black pepper. Add 1 crumbled rye crisp* instead of tortilla strips and a small side of steamed mixed broccoli, carrots, and cauliflower.

Macaroni Grill

Grilled Chicken Spiedini with mixed greens dressed with vinegar, fresh-squeezed lemon, and black pepper, topped with 1 crumbled rye crisp* and paired with green tea*.

Olive Garden

Herb-Grilled Salmon and garden fresh salad with 1 crumbled rye crisp* or chickpeas*. Dress salad with vinegar, fresh-squeezed lemon, and black pepper.

Panera Bread

Power Chicken Hummus Bowl, paired with 2 whole-grain rye crisps*.

PF Chang's

Buddha's Feast, steamed with tofu, add almonds, with 1/2 portion of brown rice. If desired, season with mustard sauce (the sauce prepared by your server at the table).

Qdoba Mexican Grill

Salad à la carte made with lettuce, grilled chicken, pico de gallo, roasted chili corn, and guacamole, paired with green tea*.

Starbucks

Protein Bistro Box (1 egg, white cheddar cheese, honey peanut butter spread, multigrain muesli bread, apples and grapes).

Increase Your Restaurant Ordering IQ

If you're going to a restaurant with no menu available online, don't be afraid to have a quick conversation with your server. Let him or her know that you're keeping it simple and that you'd prefer your food prepared with a little olive oil rather than butter, that your vegetables be steamed instead of fried or sautéed in oil, and that you want to avoid massive portions. You can even ask them to box up half of it in advance and serve you the other half. Consider asking about whole-grain options for bread or pasta, and inquire about brown rice instead of white. You'd be surprised just how accommodating they will be; remember, they work for tips! Just be kind and gracious (not demanding or condescending), and your server (and the restaurant chef) should be more than willing to work with you.

What's Next...

In the next chapter, I'll introduce the 30-Second Burn Burst Exercise Program to incorporate into your new routine. If you're over there rolling your eyes, then listen up: exercise is one of the chief ways, and quite possibly the best way, to control your weight over time. If you want to make weight loss permanent (and I know you do), then incorporating the right type of exercise into your life is a must.

But what's *not* required is being miserable while you plod away on the treadmill for hours. This program will change your perception of exercise and save you time—and you might just enjoy it. So, no more eye rolling!

In chapter 12, you will discover a clear formula for maintaining healthy weight loss for the rest of your life.

10

THE 30-SECOND BURN
BURST EXERCISE PROGRAM

Fitness—if it came in a bottle, everybody would have a great body.
—CHER

Did you know that your fat cells actually get larger from sitting too much? Seriously, your fat expands when your life is made up of a never-ending succession of various forms of seats. Have you ever heard the term "secretarial spread"? It's the idea that your rear end will spread out to fill the width of the chair you're sitting in for hours on end. No disrespect to secretaries, but that's not a pretty picture! So if your typical routine takes you from lying in bed to sitting at a desk to sitting in a car to sitting in front of a television and then back to lying in bed day after day, week after week, month after month, then I've got news for you—you're living a sedentary lifestyle. And it doesn't matter what you eat or don't eat—your body will not change for good unless and until you get up and move it.

In case you haven't noticed, the business of fitness has exploded over the past decade. From workout contraptions of every shape, size, and price point to intense at-home exercise DVDs, magazines, books, classes, and trainers, we're talking about billions of dollars paid by consumers with visions of six-pack abs or sculpted rear ends dancing in their heads. As the industry has boomed, more and more studies have been conducted to discover new exercise forms and methods that can help the human body achieve weight loss and good health. A lot of new theories have emerged and my team has used this new information to build the 30-Second Burn Burst Exercise Program. We think it's an exciting program to help you fit exercise into your busy lifestyle and keep you from getting bored.

If you're thinking, "Dr. Phil, I already go to the gym, so get off my back!" then I've got news for you. You might have spent hours at the gym on the elliptical trainer or pushing the pedals on the recumbent bike while reading your favorite novel or watching TV, barely breaking a sweat during your marathon session. What if I told you that new exercise theories suggest that you may be able to burn the same amount of calories with less time trudging away at the gym if you worked in some short bursts of high intensity? Well, get ready to be outraged (in the best possible way). Low-intensity, super-long sessions may be your opportune time for getting through a huge stack of magazines or watching your favorite TV shows, but there may be a way to get more out of your workout than catching up on the latest *Real Housewives* drama.

The truth is, some scientists believe that "long and slow" is not the best fat-burning formula. New theories regarding how the body burns off sugar and fat (both are forms of energy) suggest that when you get yourself into a high-intensity zone for short periods of time ("bursts"), you ratchet up your body's fat burning significantly. Translation: this type of exercise could help you accomplish more in less time.

So, let's get efficient.

Current Physical Activity Quiz

First, you need to identify your starting point, because it will determine how you will work yourself into the exercise plan. Answer the following questions honestly:

On average, how many hours per day do you spend in the seated position? (Take into account your commute, your work, mealtimes, watching TV or movies, etc.)

a. 6 or more hours

b. 3–5 hours

c. 1–2 hours

Given the choice, if you had to get from the first to the third floor of a building, would you be more likely to:

a. Take an elevator, no matter what. (Aren't stairs just for an emergency?)
b. Take the stairs only if I'm rushed and the elevator wasn't fast enough.
c. Take the stairs, regardless of how quickly I need to get there.

When you drive to a destination such as the mall or a grocery store, do you:

a. Circle the lot until I can park as close to the entrance as possible.
b. Park as closely to the entrance as possible, but don't spend a lot of time looking for a close spot.
c. Park far away so I can get in some extra walking.

When you're doing light activity such as vacuuming or raking the yard, how do you feel?

a. Quickly worn out; I need to take breaks every few minutes.
b. Able to do the task, but my heart rate goes up and I breathe pretty hard.
c. Strong and energized.

How often do you complete at least 20 minutes of purposeful exercise that makes you work up a sweat?

a. 1 day per week or less
b. 2–4 days per week
c. 5–7 days per week

After an average day of being awake for at least 12 hours, how do you feel?

a. Exhausted; ready to flip on the TV or crash into bed.
b. Pretty tired, but able to stay awake for a couple hours of TV time.
c. Vibrant, awake, and ready for more!

How would your heart rate be affected if you did 10 jumping jacks?

    a. My heart would probably beat right out of my chest.

    b. It would beat fast and take a few minutes to slow back down.

    c. It would speed up a little, but not much.

What is your preferred method of relaxation or stress relief?

    a. Lying on the couch or in bed reading, watching TV, etc.

    b. Mild activity such as gentle stretching, light gardening, etc.

    c. More strenuous activity such as going for a bike ride, jog, walk, etc.

Scoring

For every question that you answered "a," give yourself 0 points, for every "b" answer give yourself 2 points, and for every "c" answer, give yourself 4 points.

0 to 10: Sedentary

If your score is this low, you should not start out with the Burn Burst Exercise Program. Instead, you need to make it your immediate goal to start walking more. Walk around the room when you're on the phone, park farther away from the entrance to buildings, walk in circles around the living room while watching TV. Wherever, however, and whenever you possibly can, get on your feet and move around.

11 to 20: Mildly Active

If you're in this range, you are already making certain efforts to incorporate physical activity into your life, and I'm going to ask you to step it up a few notches. You should ease into the program below, but be extremely cognizant of your perceived exertion, which I'll explain shortly. Do not try to go from 0 to 60, but build slowly on the base you have already begun to form.

21 to 32: Active

This range indicates that you likely already understand the importance of movement in your daily life. But now we will push you even harder and use the latest research to maximize your results. Closely monitor your progress on this plan, and have an open mind as you engage in a new way of getting exercise.

Seek Your Doctor's Permission

Regardless of your current physical activity level, I am telling you in no uncertain terms that you need to discuss this exercise program with your doctor before you start it. This is not an option; it's required.

If you have any preexisting conditions that could be affected or exacerbated by activity, or if you've been extremely sedentary for a long time, then you need to take certain steps before you even attempt this program. If you don't, you might be setting yourself up for a cardiac event such as a heart attack.

This isn't just some throwaway disclaimer. If your cardiovascular system is healthy, then exercise can help maintain your health. But if it's not, then heed your doctor's advice.

Rate of Perceived Exertion (RPE)

Before we get into the specifics of this innovative form of exercise, I want you to start tuning in to your body. So many people just trudge their way through their day (or their life), barely aware of their surroundings, much less of the cues their own bodies are giving them. But when you really wake up, pay attention, and start listening, you'll be amazed how many messages your body is trying to send you.

For example, the Hunger and Fullness Scale has shown you to discern when you are *physically* hungry and when it's just fake hunger, conjured by your mind in response to some kind of trigger. You've learned about the physical symptoms you experience when you truly need food, such as a growling stomach or light-headedness. Similarly,

Get Movin' Now!

The World Health Organization and the Surgeon General recommend that adults get a minimum of 150 weekly minutes of moderate-intensity physical activity (e.g., walking, dancing, light swimming) or 75 weekly minutes of vigorous activity (e.g., running, cycling, fast swimming). If you do this you'll experience some health benefits, but for even better results and weight loss, the recommendation is to shoot for 300 minutes of moderate-intensity activity or 150 minutes of vigorous activity per week.

But if you're currently living a sedentary lifestyle, all that activity probably sounds overwhelming and unrealistic. Well, before you decide it's out of the question, here's some good news. A study in the journal *Preventive Medicine* showed that sedentary adults who complete short bouts of light to moderate physical activity (such as walking briskly around the block) for just six minutes at a time, five times per day, can experience similarly significant improvements in their overall physical fitness as people who complete one, continuous bout of exercise. You know the old joke about how to eat an elephant? One bite at a time. It's the same with exercise. You don't have to do it all at once, especially when you're first starting out.

I'd like you to become acutely aware of another set of indications, or signs, that your body is giving you on a daily basis, and these have to do with your physical exertion.

There's been quite a bit of discussion in the exercise community about whether a heart rate monitor gives you any more of an advantage than simply self-monitoring your "rate of perceived exertion" (RPE). Basically, your RPE is your built-in system for judging your own physical output. I'm talking about heavy breathing, rapid heart rate, sweat, a feeling of fatigue in major muscle groups, and so on. Your mind perceives how much you're moving, whether you're sitting as still as a statue on the couch or running full out on a treadmill.

Below is a version of an RPE scale that I have adapted from the Borg Scale of Perceived Exertion and expanded upon so that you can rate your level of energy expenditure without any extra gear like a heart monitor. This is meant to help you understand when you are "exercising" and when you are seriously *exercising*.

Judging Your Perceived Exertion

0	No movement; sitting still; neutral.
1	Extremely light exertion: Almost no sign of energy expenditure.
2	Light exertion: Very comfortable, no detectible increase in heart rate or respiration.
3	Mild exertion: Feeling slightly warm, a slight increase in breathing.
4	Medium exertion: Heart rate and respiration both noticeably higher.
5	Moderate exertion: Starting to sweat, breathing pretty hard, but still able to carry on a conversation.
6	Significant exertion: Sweating steadily, breathing is steady but hurried. Talking is getting slightly harder but is still possible.
7	Medium/high exertion: Feeling hot all over, sweat is dripping and showing through your clothes. You can maintain this level for a while, though. Your body is not screaming for you to stop.
8	Hard exertion: Starting to feel uncomfortable, but you feel like you can go for a few more minutes like this.
9	Intense exertion: You don't feel like you can maintain this level very long. You can get out a couple words if you have to, but definitely not a conversation.
10	Extremely intense exertion: Very heavy breathing, heart rate is extremely high, and you cannot speak. The hardest you've ever pushed yourself physically—so much so that you can't keep it up another second.

Keep in mind that you may not experience the same signals of exertion as someone else. For instance, a marathon runner would likely be at a 1 or 2 when walking briskly, while someone who isn't in shape would be at a 5 or 6 when walking at the same pace. That's why this is an ideal method to determine *your* exertion, because it's tailor-made to you and it will change and evolve as you increase your level of daily physical activity.

When I first started doing the high-intensity exercise bursts you will soon read about, I found out very quickly that you don't just go from 0 to 10 in one swift shake of your tail feathers. It takes serious labor to work your way up this scale. So, when you start to learn about the burn bursts in this program, keep in mind that your 30-second clock doesn't start ticking until you've reached an 8 or 9 on the RPE scale, and it may take you a couple minutes to get up there.

For me, the best way to apply this exercise regimen is on a stationary bicycle. I just keep increasing that resistance so it gets harder and harder to pedal and I can get into my high-intensity range. Boy, I'll tell you

Anaerobic and Aerobic Exercise

You've probably heard of aerobic exercise. Now we often refer to it as "cardio," but you might remember the days of aerobics classes. Essentially, aerobic activity occurs in the presence of oxygen, and it uses both glucose and fat for fuel. Anaerobic exercise, however, does not need oxygen—instead, it uses glycogen, which is the sugar stored in your muscles, as its fuel. This type of activity builds muscle tissue, which we know to be metabolically active and excellent at burning fat. When you perform the type of high-intensity interval training I'm suggesting in this chapter, the 30-second bursts are considered anaerobic activity.

So, which type of exercise is best for burning off fat and calories? Both! This Burn Burst Exercise Program combines aerobic and anaerobic activity to help you lose weight and build muscle.

what: if I sat down on the bike cold and tried to move those pedals at that resistance level, I couldn't do much more than stand on them! My point is, you've got to first let yourself work your way up the RPE scale and *then* start timing your "burst" when you reach an 8 or 9.

Before we launch into the specifics of the exercise program, I'd like to remind you—these routines will not take that much time out of your day. You can complete them in about 30 minutes.

Cardio Burn Bursts

The official term for this type of cardiovascular exercise is HIIT, which stands for High-Intensity Interval Training. The basic concept is that you're completing short bursts of intense exercise (an 8, 9, or even a 10 on the RPE scale) and then immediately returning to a recovery pace for a slightly longer period of time before starting the next burst of intensity. If your exercise sessions were plotted out on a graph, you would see peaks and valleys rather than just one steady pace across time. A growing body of research suggests that this sort of high-intensity, low-volume interval training is an efficient form of exercise.

One potential benefit of this type of exercise is that it can save you time. Some studies in this area suggest that, by varying the intensity of your workout, you can accomplish more for your body in less time. More research is needed to confirm this effect, as many of the studies so far have been small and had other limitations, but the most important thing is that I'm getting you off the couch and moving.

I was convinced by these potential benefits so I gave it a shot, and I've been very impressed with the results in my body. I have more energy overall, I perform better on the tennis court, and my physical fitness has improved.

This form of exercise might be a new concept for you, so I want you to pay very close attention to your body's signals. Obviously, don't push so hard during the 30-second bursts that you pass out or otherwise can't complete the workout. But I want you to reap the most benefits, so find that "sweet spot" of pure energy expenditure. You'll quickly adapt and, call me crazy, but very soon you will find this exhilarating. You will experience a rush of endorphins, a certain powerful chemical in your brain, which can make you feel happier and even euphoric. You've probably heard of the term "runner's high," and it was coined because of these feel-good chemicals that exercise naturally helps your body release. Stick to this workout and you'll start to look forward to and even crave exercise.

Cardio Burn Burst Exercise Routine

Complete the following workout two to three times a week on days when you do not do any resistance training, which I'll tell you about shortly.

Warm up with light cardio for three to five minutes.
Examples of light cardio:

- Brisk walking
- Slow jogging
- Dancing
- Jumping jacks

Start your 30-second burn burst cycle.

Choose a cardio activity to which you have access, whether in your home, at the gym, or outdoors. Do it full out, high intensity, for 30 seconds.

Note: Your 30 seconds START when you reach an 8 or 9 on the RPE scale. It will take you at least a few seconds, and maybe even a minute, before you reach that level of exertion. When you're there, start timing. If you cannot sustain this pace for 30 full seconds, just go as long as you can, and keep track each time because as you continue to exercise in this way, you will find that you're able to go a little longer each session.

Slow down for 60 to 90 seconds with that same cardio activity (recovery pace).
Allow your heart rate and breathing to slow, but be careful not to return all the way to a resting pace, or else the next burst will be much harder.

Start your next 30-second burn burst.

As before, you'll need at least a few seconds to reach an 8 or 9 on the RPE scale. When you reach it, begin timing. Keep up that pace for as long as you can, but not more than 30 seconds.

Slow down to a recovery pace.

Repeat this sequence 8 times, for a total of 8 burn bursts and 8 recoveries. The total workout time will be around 15 to 20 minutes.

Note: Depending on your starting level of fitness, you may want to start with 2 to 4 burn bursts. But in subsequent weeks, as your body catches on to your new regimen, you should increase burn bursts until you can do 10 to 12 in a session.

Resistance Burn Bursts

Exercise isn't nearly as effective or efficient if you ignore resistance training. It's the combination of cardio *and* resistance that can help you get a toned, overall healthy body. This is why I want you to integrate this resistance program into your overall exercise plan.

The official name for this type of exercise is HIRT, which stands for High-intensity Interval Resistance Training.

To do this, you'll need some light weights (you might want to start at 1- to 2-pound hand weights if you're brand new to weightlifting) or resistance bands. Many trainers and fitness professionals recommend resistance bands, especially for beginners. They're very inexpensive, easy to use, and they pack easily so you have no excuse not to exercise while you're traveling.

This is a type of circuit training, in which you'll pair different moves with noncompeting muscle groups, such as a lower body exercise and an upper body exercise, with only 30 seconds between sets. These are called compound exercises, and some scientists believe that they are very effective at burning fat and building lean muscle mass.

For example, you'll do a set of 8 to 10 Sumo Squats, which work your inner and outer thighs, and then immediately (no rest between) complete a Bicycle Move, which works your abs and core, and *then* take a 30-second rest before moving on to the next paired set.

Be reasonable and do not endanger yourself by using weights that are too heavy or trying to get through a workout that is hurting in all the wrong places. Ease yourself into this and be smart.

The Resistance Burn Burst Moves

Now let's get into the types of HIRT moves you'll be completing in this exercise routine. Take a close look at these and make sure you really understand them before you dive in. On the free 20/20 Diet app, you will find videos showing you exactly how to do each of these moves with proper form.

Again, you will need either hand weights or a resistance band for many of these moves, but start light if this is brand new to you. You can work yourself up to heavier weights over time.

Here are clear explanations of the various moves you will be performing in this HIRT workout.

Walking Lunges (works the thighs, hamstrings, glutes, and calves)

Begin with your legs together and feet planted firmly on the floor. Step forward about 1½ to 2 feet on your right foot. Bend your right knee so that your right thigh is parallel with the floor, at a 90-degree angle. Your left (back) knee should be bent, nearly touching the floor. Return to the starting position by standing up and repeat with the left leg. Keep lunging forward, alternating legs. Do this 8 to 10 times.

Note: Make sure your lunging knee does not extend out past your ankle.

Dumbbell Rows (works the back)

Place your left knee on an exercise bench or the seat of a sturdy chair. Bend your torso forward so that it is parallel to the floor. Take a dumbbell in your right hand and keep your right arm straight. Bend your right elbow and pull the weight up toward your side, keeping your arm close to your side. Lower and repeat for 8 to 10 repetitions. Repeat the exercise on the other side.

Note: Make sure your back remains straight during this move.

Squats (works the thighs and glutes)

Begin with your feet about shoulder-width apart, holding a dumbbell in each hand and with your arms by your sides. Bend your knees and lower your torso so that your thighs are as close to parallel to the floor as you can get them. Keep your back as straight as possible and your chest up so that you can see yourself if you're looking in a mirror. Slowly return to the starting position. Repeat 8 to 10 times.

Note: Stay erect and centered as you descend. Do not allow your knees to extend forward and go out past your ankles.

Chest Press (works the pectoral muscles/chest)

Lie on your back on a flat exercise bench or soft floor surface. Take a dumbbell in each hand and hold the weights at the sides of your chest with elbows bent. Press the dumbbells straight up to a position just over your chest, with your arms straight. Purposely contract your chest muscles at the top of the movement. Slowly lower the dumbbells to the starting position. Repeat 8 to 10 times.

Note: Do not use a weight that is too heavy here; you don't want to drop it when your hands are directly over your face!

Sumo Squats (works the inner and outer thighs)

Stand with your feet wider than shoulder width and your toes pointed out at a 45-degree angle. Hold a dumbbell in each hand, keeping your arms down by your sides. Bend your knees and lower your torso so that your thighs are as close to parallel to the floor as possible, while holding your chest up. Keep your back straight. Slowly return to the starting position. Repeat 8 to 10 times.

Note: If you notice any knee pain, do not go as deep into this move.

Bicycle Move (works the core/abdominal muscles)

Lie on your back on the floor. Place your hands behind your head and bend your knees to a 45-degree angle to the floor, with your feet in the air. Lift your shoulders off the floor slightly. Bring your opposite knee (left knee, for example) to your opposite elbow (right elbow, in this example) and simultaneously straighten out the other leg. Alternate legs and elbows for this exercise. Continue the exercise for as many reps as you can, up to 50 at a time.

Note: Continue to draw your belly button in toward your spine during this move rather than letting your belly pooch out.

Chest Fly (works the pectoral muscles/chest)

Grasp a dumbbell in each hand and lie on your back on a weight bench or an ottoman, with the dumbbells resting on your chest. Stretch your arms out to the side and bend your elbows slightly. Raise your arms up in an arc, over your chest, until your hands meet at the top (palms facing toward each other). Contract your chest muscles. Slowly lower to the starting position and repeat 8 to 10 times. Be sure to select a dumbbell weight you can lift comfortably.

Calf Raise (works the calves)

Stand on a stair or raised platform so that your toes are on and your heels are off the surface. Hold on to a sturdy object (e.g., the stair railing; a chair) with one hand for balance. Raise up on your toes as high as you can, then slowly lower down, stretching your calf muscles. Continue raising and lowering your feet in this manner for 16 to 20 repetitions.

Shoulder Press with a Resistance Band (works the shoulders)

Stand on the middle of the resistance band with your feet about shoulder-width apart. Hold the handles, facing your palms forward. Stretch the band upward and hold the handles at your shoulders in a bent-arm position (like a standard biceps curl). Then, raise the band straight up and straighten your elbows at the top of the movement. Slowly lower the band to the starting position and repeat 8 to 10 times.

Note: Continue to pull your arms in as you press the band upward so they are directly on either side of your head as you do this move.

Seated Reverse Crunch (works the core/abdominal muscles)

Sit on a chair or a flat workout bench, close to its edge. Grasp the sides of the chair or bench with your hands and lean backward slightly, keeping your back straight. Bend your knees and pull them in toward your chest. Next, extend your legs straight out in front of you. Return to the starting position and continue the exercise for as many reps as you can, up to 50 at a time.

Note: Continue to draw your belly button in toward your spine during this move rather than letting your belly pooch out.

Push-ups (works the chest, triceps, and core/abdominal muscles)

Lie facedown on an exercise mat (the floor works fine if you don't have one) with your hands placed flat on the mat on either side of your chest. Keep your toes pointed downward into the mat. Press up on your hands, lifting your body off the mat. Straighten your arms at the top of the movement. Keep your back straight and parallel to the floor and your eyes looking forward so that your head does not droop. Slowly lower to the starting position. Continue for 8 to 10 repetitions.

Note: You may also do this exercise from a knees-bent position rather than from your toes.

Biceps Curl with a Resistance Band (works the biceps)

Stand on the middle of the band with your feet about shoulder-width apart. Hold the handles with your palms facing away from your body and your arms straight down at your sides. Flex your elbows and bring the band up toward your chest in a curl motion, making sure that your elbows remain fixed against your body. Slowly lower the band to the starting position and repeat 8 to 10 times.

Note: Purposely contract the bicep muscles when you bring your arms up.

Dumbbell Deadlift (works the glutes, back, and hamstrings)

Place two dumbbells on the floor in front of your feet. Begin with your feet about shoulder-width apart, with your knees slightly bent. Bend your knees and, keeping your back straight and chest up, pick up both dumbbells. Slowly stand up to the starting position, squeezing your glute (butt) muscles tightly at the top position. Pull your shoulder blades together as you squeeze. Lower slowly, following the same path you used to lift the weights. Continue this movement for 8 to 10 repetitions.

Triceps Press with a Resistance Band (works the triceps)

Stand on the middle of the band with your feet about shoulder-width apart. Take the handles and hold your palms facing forward. Lift your arms and hold them at your shoulders in a bent-arm position. Press upward to an overhead position so that your hands meet behind your head, but don't let your elbows drift out to the sides—they should be extending forward at this point. Straighten your arms all the way to a full extension, as if opening your elbows like a hinge. Flex your triceps at the top of the exercise, and then slowly lower until your hands are back behind your head. Repeat 8 to 10 times.

Dips (works the triceps)

Position your body so that your back is facing the edge of a bench, ottoman, or sturdy chair. With both hands, grasp the edge of the object with your hands; your palms should be facing downward and your fingers forward, toward your back. Your elbows should be bent slightly to start. Extend your legs out in front of you. Using the strength of your arms, straighten your triceps to a locked-out position, lifting your body upward slightly. Slowly lower to the starting position and repeat the exercise 8 to 10 times.

The Resistance Burn Burst Exercise Routine

This workout should take about 30 to 45 minutes to perform, and you should work up to doing it a total of three days per week on nonconsecutive days so you give your muscles time to recover properly. The idea is to keep the rest period between moves to 30 seconds or less. That's the intensity part of the high-intensity workout. By not letting your body fully recover between sets, you are boosting the overall calorie burn.

Warm-up: 5 minutes light cardio.

Walking Lunges/Dumbbell Rows—8 to 10 reps each exercise

30-second rest

Squats/Chest Press—8 to 10 reps each exercise

30-second rest

Sumo Squats/Bicycle Move—8 to 10 times for the Sumo Squat; up to 50 reps for the Bicycle Move

30-second rest

Chest Fly/Calf Raise on Platform or Stairs—8 to 10 reps for the Chest Fly; 16 to 20 reps for the Calf Raises

30-second rest

Shoulder Press/Seated Reverse Crunch—8 to 10 reps for the Shoulder Press; up to 50 reps for the Reverse Crunch

30-second rest

Push-ups/Biceps Curl—8 to 10 reps each exercise

30-second rest

Dumbbell Deadlift/Triceps Press or Dips—8 to 10 reps each exercise

Once you have two or three weeks of this routine under your belt, start working on repeating each set. Doubling up will increase the speed of your progress.

Program Your New Active Lifestyle

In *The Ultimate Weight Solution*, I talked about how you should program your life for your new level of activity. Likewise, here are the important steps you need to take in order to make this new exercise regimen just another part of your overall routine:

1. Recognize the Payoffs of Exercise

The benefits of exercise in any weight loss program are numerous. Exercise has the power to improve overall health and appearance. You need to internalize these benefits so you know why you are making this effort.

2. Make It Motivating

These burst training routines can be done almost anywhere, with varying types of activities, so choose a place and type that appeal to you. If you enjoy companionship while exercising, get a friend, family member, or coworker to join you. For example, start a walking group at work or in the neighborhood. And here's a tip: listen to music that motivates you during your workout. Studies show that you're more likely to move or walk faster if you're listening to upbeat music.

3. "Consequate" Your Exercise Behavior

If you currently find exercise less than desirable, pair it with a positive reward so that in order to get the reward, you must first exercise. For example, you might tell your kids they cannot watch TV until they do their homework. (If they don't do their homework, the consequence is no TV.) Similarly, find something, anything, that you will not allow yourself to do *until* you've exercised each day. It could be combing your hair, reading the newspaper, taking a shower—anything that you value and want/need to do.

4. Monitor Your Progress

You started this program with 20/20 vision about what your future would look like when you slim down because it will help propel you to your finish line. Every step of the way, you've got to take mental or physical notes of how you're improving each week. If you are using the RPE scale, take note of how long it takes you to get to an 8 or 9 on the scale. That time will start to decrease. Also, take a full-body photo of yourself before you start the program and then more photos every couple of weeks so you can look back and see the change in your muscles and physique. You might even modify your vision of the future as you see what you're capable of and remind yourself that your hard work leads to definitive and measurable progress.

Reducing Muscle Soreness

Anytime you start a new exercise program that your body isn't used to, you are going to experience some soreness in your muscles. Look at it as a positive sign that you are putting those muscles to work so they can work even harder for you as you progress. Your body will adapt to this program, and you won't get as sore as you continue it.

Here's a word to the wise: as with the cardio portion of this program, make sure that when you are in the recovery period between 30-second high-intensity bursts, you are not stopping activity altogether. You must keep going so that you're at least hitting a 5 or 6 on the RPE scale. Research indicates that this helps your body reduce the lactic acid buildup in your muscles faster than if you were just to stop completely between bursts.

Putting It All Together

Once you're ready to start this entire program, your first step is to map out what you'll be doing each day of the week. You should even prescribe a set time for each workout so that it's in your calendar and on your mind. It's not just your long-term goal that requires 20/20 vision; you've got to have a schedule for every day and the overall week so you know exactly how you will work exercise into your daily routine; then you will be far more likely to actually do it.

Leaving your exercise to chance and thinking "I'll do it when I have time" is too risky. Something always comes up, and it's so easy to convince yourself that the "something" takes precedence over your exercise. Instead, you have to look at this time as sacred. This is *your* time, for *your* health, and no one is stealing that from you because you are setting up boundaries around this time.

I did this in my own life years ago. Everyone understands that I play tennis in the afternoons. During that time, I am unavailable for anything else. Period. If I didn't cordon off this time for my exercise, there's no doubt that someone would take up that hour of my day. It's true in all of our lives; someone will always need or want something from us. But unless it's a true emergency, you need to give yourself permission to be selfish and stop using the needs of others as your excuse for neglecting the physical needs of your own body.

This might mean waking up earlier so you can work out before your day begins. Or you might need to DVR your evening TV show so you can exercise at a time when you're normally nestling down in the couch cushions while munching popcorn (which shouldn't be part of your evening routine anymore anyway!).

Use this space to create your first week of an exercise schedule that makes sense for you. Make sure you are giving yourself one rest day per week. On the 20/20 Diet app, you can create workout calendars and even set reminders for upcoming workouts.

Day of the Week	Type of Workout	# of 30-Second Bursts	✔ When Complete
Monday			
Tuesday			
Wednesday			
Thursday			
Friday			
Saturday			
Sunday			

This plan can help you change the way you perceive exercise. As you increase your strength and endurance, you'll see and feel the results. Make this a part of your life now and enjoy the benefits for years to come when you incorporate exercise into your routine as a life-long habit.

11

WHEN YOUR BODY WON'T FOLLOW YOUR MIND:

ARE YOU RESISTANT TO WEIGHT LOSS?

Never confuse a single defeat with a final defeat.
—F. Scott Fitzgerald

When it comes to failed weight loss attempts, there are generally two types of people. There are those who know, deep down, that they haven't lost the weight and kept it off as a direct result of something they're doing or not doing. These folks make poor choices: they eat in response to emotion, they don't stick to a plan for any reasonable amount of time, they lie to themselves, they make excuses, and so on. They know that if they would just put in the effort and do what was required of them, they could lose the weight.

Then there are those people who really, truly commit to eating healthy, exercising, and living a lifestyle that should, for all intents and purposes, lend itself to achieving a healthy weight. But no matter how hard they try, their weight simply will not budge. When you know—and I mean deep down in your gut *know*—that you're doing everything by the book, you're conducting yourself and your life in such a way that the only logical outcome is weight loss, but the scale continues to tell a very different story, you feel frustrated, defeated, confused, and downright ticked off.

In *The Ultimate Weight Solution*, I discussed the concept of weight loss resistance. Back then it was a very new notion, and not one that was widely accepted. Since then, doctors and weight loss experts have conducted more studies on weight loss resistance. It is real, it is recognized by weight loss professionals, and they now have a much better understanding of weight loss resistance and its various root causes.

So, if you've been putting in the hard work that's necessary for years but your weight loss attempts have just felt like an endless series of banging your head against the same wall, hear me now. You're *not* crazy. Weight loss resistance is a description for an entire category of people who, due to certain physiological imbalances, are unable to lose fat through traditional methods of healthy diet and regular exercise.

The causes range from thyroid malfunction to hormone imbalance, sleep deprivation to food intolerances or digestive imbalance, and more. Because there are many potential sources of the problem, there isn't a one-size-fits-all treatment that works for all weight loss resistant individuals. The key is to uncover your own, specific chemical imbalance or physiological "glitch" so that your doctor can target it with a treatment plan tailored to you. Until you talk to your doctor, you cannot be sure what plan is best for you, including if the plan in this book would help you lose weight. And thanks to all the research conducted on the subject in recent years, doctors are armed with more methods for you to manage and treat the core of your problem than ever before.

As I revealed earlier in this book, I identify with what you've been going through on a very personal level. Having been an athlete for my entire life, it was more than a little alarming when I found, a few years ago, that I was struggling to maintain my target, healthy weight. I was moving in what felt like slow motion across the tennis court in my afternoon games and feeling winded far too easily. The subtle signs started to add up, and despite my efforts to push myself harder physically and becoming hyperaware of my food intake, my body simply said, "Sorry, buddy, but you're wasting your time here. Something is off." So I pursued the medical experts for answers.

It turned out that I have metabolic syndrome, a genetic disposition that was transmitted to me from my father. The tests revealed that my triglycerides were sky high, as was my blood sugar, and to top it all off, I had insulin resistance, so I was not processing sugar properly. My body was just hanging on to absolutely everything I put in it and not letting go. I simply wasn't configured for weight loss.

The good news for me, and for you if you fit the bill, is that all of this is manageable with the right nutritional and medical plan. I got started right away working with my doctors to get my blood sugars stabilized and bring everything back into proper balance so my body would start releasing the weight again. But this experience was about much more than just my weight. I shudder to think where I might be now had I not jumped right on this problem, because I was unwittingly on the road to some devastating illnesses, including heart disease. Now that I've learned, with the help of my doctor, how to manage my body chemistry, my weight has remained in a safe range and I am healthier overall. The very same can happen for you if you talk to your doctor.

I really want you to get this: You are not destined to be overweight or obese just because you got a raw deal in the metabolic or biochemical department. You do not have to feel trapped in your body anymore. I know you'd do anything to get out of the quicksand and onto dry land and win back control over your weight. I'm extending you a helping hand, so read carefully because it's more than just your weight we're talking about now. It's your life.

Identifying Signs of Weight Loss Resistance

If all of this is resonating with you and you have serious concerns that there could be a physiological cause for your inability to lose weight, then the first order of business is to closely examine your symptoms so that you can present them to your physician.

To get you started on your internal inspection, here is a list of some common symptoms to discuss with your medical professional because they might indicate weight loss resistance. But, just remember this is not an exhaustive list and if you are experiencing any physical issues that you are worried about, you should bring them to your doctor's attention.

- Do you find yourself unable to lose weight, despite closely following a healthy eating plan and exercise program?

- Has your physician diagnosed you with or medicated you for three or more of these conditions: high triglycerides (150 or higher), low HDL cholesterol (less than 50), high blood pressure, or elevated blood sugar?

- Do you experience gastrointestinal symptoms such as diarrhea, constipation, acid reflux, nausea, vomiting, or bloating two times or more per month? Or, do you notice any of these digestive symptoms or headaches after eating wheat, dairy, soy, eggs, or nut products?

- Is your natural waist measurement (the area 1 inch above your belly button) 35 inches or more if you're a woman, or 40 inches or more if you are a man?

- Have you recently been experiencing disruptive sleep patterns such as waking up often during the night or finding it difficult to fall asleep, or do you sleep six or fewer hours most nights of the week?

- Are you feeling any of these symptoms: increased sensitivity to cold, drastic changes in your body temperature, thinning hair, excessively dry skin, hoarseness, memory loss, or difficulty concentrating?

- Have you recently been under chronic (ongoing) stress in your life? The kind of stress that you cannot seem to resolve? Take a moment here to measure your stress level on a scale from 1 to 5, with 5 being the highest level of stress and 1 being the lowest. Is your stress level 3 or higher?

- Are you on any of these medications: antidepressants, diabetes medications, steroids, blood pressure medications, antiseizure drugs, sleeping pills, birth control, or any form of hormone replacement therapy (HRT)?

- Do you use or abuse illicit drugs or abuse prescription medications that have not been prescribed to you?

- Women only: Have you been told by a doctor that you are menopausal or perimenopausal, or have you ever been diagnosed with polycystic ovary syndrome? Or are you often experiencing two or more of these symptoms: hot flashes, mood swings, tender breasts, vaginal dryness, excessive sweating, or changes in menstruation?

You cannot know with certainty if you fall into this weight loss resistance category without a medical evaluation because everyone's body chemistry is different. There are specific tests that can give your doctor the data needed to properly diagnose you and create a treatment plan, but the idea is to be an informed patient by asking the right questions and providing the right information when you visit your doctor.

Collecting Data

When I visited the doctor with my initial concerns, I didn't just plop down on the exam table and say, "Hey Doc, I can't lose weight. Fix me." Instead, I did my homework and provided my doctor with the whole picture. No one knows my body better than me, and no one knows yours better than you. So, be your own advocate by telling your physician the whole story.

Your whole story includes any of the symptoms above, any other symptoms you are concerned about, as well as a complete list of all the vitamins, supplements, and medications you're taking because they could affect the way your body functions or the way it stores food. They might not seem significant to you, but your doctor could very well spot something on your list that's a potential culprit.

You should also bring a food journal like the one you filled out in chapter 3, or at least a list of foods you've been eating often or any new foods you've recently started eating. This may tip off your doctor to any food sensitivities or contraindications of certain foods with certain medications. You might have developed (or always had) a dairy intolerance, for example, and the simple act of removing dairy products from your life could help you get rid of bloating. Include in

Checklist: What to Share with Your Doctor

Symptom List:
- Anything from the list we just discussed
- Other symptoms, even if you don't *think* they relate to weight loss

Medication/Supplement List:
- Prescription medications (and dosages)
- Over-the-counter medications you often take (and dosages)
- Vitamins, minerals, and supplements
- Herbs (and dosages)
- Illicit drugs or medical marijuana

Food/Drink Journal:
- Foods and drinks (including alcohol) you commonly consume
- Any new foods or drinks you've recently added

Exercise Pattern:
- Amount and type of physical activity you're getting in a week

Chronic Stress:
- Any new or ongoing causes of stress

Sleep Patterns:
- Amount and quality of sleep you're getting every night

this list your current alcohol intake, even if it's just a glass of wine in the evenings, because that can play a role. And if you are using medicinal marijuana or illicit drugs, you need to be honest with your doctor about that too. Everything you're consuming could be an important clue in your weight loss mystery.

Another critical factor you need to share with your physician is your current activity level. If you used to be a three times per week gym-goer, but in the last few months you've called a cease-fire on all exercise because you can barely drag yourself up a flight of stairs, much less work out, that's significant. Or if you've amped up your exercise to a frenzied pace in a desperate attempt to move the needle on the scale, that's important too.

Chronic stress can have a substantial effect on your biochemistry and is definitely something to discuss with your physician. Stress comes in many forms, but it is insidious and it can ravage your organs and bodily functions. If you're living each day as though you're a rat in a maze with no exit, there's no doubt that stress is taking a physical toll. Bring it up so your doctor can inspect you for adrenal fatigue and other physical symptoms of chronic stress.

Sleep is also a key piece to this puzzle. Have you had problems sleeping lately? Do you take sleeping medications regularly? Are you hardly ever getting seven to nine hours of sleep per night? Are you sleeping too much? Tell your doctor if you have experienced any irregularities in your sleeping patterns. It may help to write down your sleep pattern for two to three nights in a row before you go in.

Now let's talk in a little more depth about a few common causes of weight loss resistance and the diagnostic tools used to identify them. I want you to be well informed about these causes, but this information in no way substitutes for the opinion of your doctor. It is imperative that if you think a medical problem is making it difficult to lose weight, that you talk to your physician.

Metabolic Syndrome

According to guidelines set by the American Heart Association, when you have three or more of the following factors, you have metabolic syndrome: high blood pressure, high blood sugar, excess visceral fat (an accumulation of fat around your belly area), and abnormal cholesterol levels (such as low HDL or high triglycerides). This puts you in a higher risk category for some dangerous illnesses, including type 2 diabetes, cardiovascular disease, stroke, some cancers, liver disease, and more.

If you think you are in this category, then there are some tests you need to request from your physician. But first there is one test you can do on your own. In chapter 4, I asked you to take an accurate waist measurement. If you're a woman and your waist measures 35 inches or more, or if you're a man and it measures 40 inches or more, you have *one* of the conditions for metabolic syndrome.

The tests you should request from your doctor are as follows:

- **Fasting blood glucose:** This test determines how much glucose (a certain type of sugar) you have in your blood.

- **Triglycerides:** This is typically part of your overall cholesterol panel, and it measures the amount of triglycerides (a type of fat) you have in your blood.

- **HDL:** Also a typical part of your overall cholesterol panel, it measures the amount of HDL (your "good" cholesterol, which helps remove your "bad" cholesterol) in your blood.

- **Blood pressure:** These days you can even get your blood pressure checked at a number of local pharmacies, so there's really no excuse for not knowing if you have high blood pressure.

Like me, you might have inherited some of these factors. It's frustrating, but guess what? Life isn't fair, so get used to it! These conditions can all be managed with your doctor's assistance and the right treatment plan. Once you get your numbers back into the healthy range, your body will be properly configured for weight loss again.

If it was your weight problem that actually caused these issues in the first place, that doesn't mean you're out of luck. You might need the assistance of medication (perhaps temporarily) in combination with your new healthy eating and exercise plan as prescribed by your doctor. Bottom line: have the tests, talk to your doctor about your concerns, create a clear plan of attack, and more than anything, don't give up!

Thyroid Hormone Imbalance

When your thyroid hormones go haywire, you could experience all kinds of symptoms, including changes in your body temperature, fatigue, hair loss, hoarseness, changes in texture of your skin, memory issues, and more. If your thyroid gland isn't firing on all cylinders, then you might also start to pack on the pounds because your thyroid is responsible for regulating your metabolism. Don't ignore any of these symptoms, and by all means, discuss them with your doctor.

If your physician thinks you may have an underactive thyroid, he or she will order tests such as a thyroid ultrasound (to inspect the physical structure of the gland and to see if there are any goiters) and blood tests to check your thyroid hormone levels.

Should your test results indicate a problem with the function of your thyroid, there are specific treatments you can undergo, and very often, once the medications get your thyroid back up and running properly, your metabolism will normalize and the excess weight will start to come off.

Estrogen Imbalance

If you're a woman and you are perimenopausal, menopausal, on hormone replacement therapy, have taken birth control pills for years, or have been diagnosed with polycystic ovary syndrome, it's very possible that your female hormones, especially your estrogen, are imbalanced, which could lead to weight problems. Some symptoms that could indicate a hormonal imbalance are mood swings, tender breasts, fluctuations in menstruation, genital dryness, hot flashes, or excessive sweating.

There is a lot of information floating around on the Internet about female hormones. As with all of these medical conditions, do not try to self-diagnose. It's important that you go to a gynecologist or general physician whose opinion you trust and discuss your symptoms and suspicions. Don't jump to conclusions or try to take matters into your own hands and treat yourself with herbs and supplements. A doctor should guide your treatment plan if a hormonal imbalance is the cause of your body's refusal to lose weight.

Sleep Disorders

The lack of good sleep can totally derail your weight loss efforts. Sleep deprivation can lead to more hunger throughout the day, and studies show that sleep-deprived people consume more calories on a daily basis.

There are two key hunger-related hormones called leptin and ghrelin that are affected by your sleep patterns. If you're not able to sleep seven to nine hours per night, those hormones can get out of sync and cause you to feel hungrier or less satisfied at meal times.

Sleep problems can also increase your risk of insulin resistance, which basically means that your body produces insulin but isn't using it properly. Insulin resistance can lead to diabetes if it's not caught early.

If you have been having trouble falling asleep or if you're waking up several times a night, you need to discuss this with your doctor. There are several underlying causes of sleep problems, ranging from stress to sleep apnea. Treatment options depend on what's at the root of your sleep issues.

Stress Fat/Cortisol Overproduction

Chronic, unresolved stress can wreak havoc on your entire body and all of its organ functions, and it has the power to block your weight loss. When you let stress run amok, it has the ability to put you into a continuous state of fight or flight. That means certain stress hormones (cortisol and adrenaline) are being pumped into your system so much that it begins to negatively impact many of your body's most basic functions.

If you think chronic stress has a choke hold on your mind and body, your doctor can help. It might be a matter of learning to manage the stress through simple cognitive-behavioral exercises, or certain medications could help even out your brain chemistry. Regardless, do not let another day pass without seeking medical guidance.

Digestive Tract Imbalance

If you're regularly faced with digestive symptoms such as bloating, acid reflux, nausea, diarrhea, constipation, or abdominal pain or discomfort, especially in connection with specific foods, you might have developed some food intolerances or sensitivities that are contributing to weight issues. It's also possible that you have an imbalance of your intestinal bacteria, which can occur for many reasons, including as a reaction to the use of antibiotics or nutritional insufficiencies. Or you might be suffering from an ulcer or GERD (gastroesophageal reflux disease), which can significantly affect your eating patterns.

Digestive symptoms can be extremely disruptive to your life, and they can also be a source of embarrassment. But your doctor can do several tests to determine what's causing your digestive distress (the tests depend upon your specific symptoms) and get you back on track with the right medication. Probiotics have been a life-changing treatment for many people, but talk to your doctor before you begin using any over-the-counter probiotics.

If food intolerances or sensitivities are found to be the source of your gastrointestinal distress, your doctor might recommend removing certain foods from your diet. If any of those foods are ones included in this diet plan, by all means, heed the advice of your doctor! In the Allergy Alert in chapter 7, you'll find a concise list of alternatives for foods in my plan that are commonly associated with intolerances.

Taking Action

Now that you have a glimpse into some of the common causes of weight loss resistance, don't just smile, nod, and then promptly ignore all of it. If medical testing and your physician's expertise reveal that you do, in fact, fall within the category of the weight loss resistant, I am telling you that it's not the end of the world. In fact, it's an important first step to becoming "weight loss triumphant" because you will finally learn the proper ways to manage your unique biochemical configuration. You can, at last, win control over your weight. You should feel lighter already now that the yokes of guilt and shame have been removed from your shoulders.

On the other hand, I want to put you on high alert for a certain reaction you might have if you find out you are not currently configured for weight loss. If you learn that your issues are, for example, inherited, then your knee-jerk reaction might be to just give up the ghost. "Well, it was just meant to be, I guess. I'm going to be fat for the rest of my life just like my parents, and if I die young, then I might as well go out with a beer in my hand and a pizza in my lap." That attitude doesn't cut it, not even close. Just because a few genetic cards are stacked against you, that doesn't mean you quit playing the game. This is when you get busy; this is the time you put your health on project status and you reprioritize so you can focus on doing whatever it takes to bring the balance back. There's really no excuse—others in your position have done it, so you can too.

No matter what treatment plan you'll now be following in order to achieve that balance, you've got to give your body time to reconfigure itself. Change doesn't happen overnight, so don't get frustrated if the fat doesn't instantly start melting like butter on hot toast. It's very likely that your body will go into temporary shock when you make a change. That's a function of our ability to survive; when homeostasis is disrupted, our bodies want to hang on to all the fat in case there are long, starving days ahead. Your body *can* learn that it doesn't need to go into starvation mode and store everything it's given, but it'll take a little while as you work through your prescribed treatment plan. You may have to work a little harder and have some patience, but good days *are* ahead. Your decision to seek medical support will be a game changer.

Remember, winners do things losers aren't willing to, and you're a winner.

12

MAINTAINING YOUR SUCCESS:
THE MANAGEMENT PHASE

*I don't want you to keep accepting what life deals up rather
than working to get what you want, need, and deserve.*
—DR. PHIL McGRAW

Weight loss success is not a one-time, fleeting moment of achievement that fades into the background of your life. Overcoming a weight problem, no matter how big or small that problem was, is a *daily* achievement. Think about it this way: When you graduate from high school or college, walk across the stage, and accept your diploma, that's thrilling, right? It's something you never forget because you're proud of your accomplishment. But it is also final because it represents the end of a journey.

Not so when it comes to weight loss. When you step on that scale and finally see a healthy number, one that you haven't seen in a long time, if ever, it's exhilarating, and I want you to take pride in that victory. *You* did that! You won the battle. But you shouldn't think of this achievement as "final." Your weight loss is an ongoing journey, one that you live every day. I don't want you to take it for granted, or else you run the risk of feeling invincible, like you can go back to all your bad behaviors without gaining back the weight.

By the time you arrive at the Management Phase of this diet, you will have formed many healthy habits and you will have developed a healthier relationship with food, so maintaining your healthy weight should be easier for you now than it was before. But you need to guard against the various danger zones and traps that can ruin everything you've done to this point. Later in this chapter, I will help you "see around corners" by identifying those common pitfalls so you can avoid them.

The Management Phase is a way of eating and living that you can truly do for the rest of your life. Because you've already spent a number of days eating healthy meal portions spaced over the span of your day, and you've familiarized yourself with your hunger signals, you are starting to feel like you're on autopilot. Your body is used to this new way of eating, and if you continue to pay attention to your needs, you can keep yourself on track without having to obsessively think about food.

What Now?

The first order of business after you've completed Phase 3 is to record your weight and measurements in chapter 4. If you have reached your goals, it's time to move on to the Management Phase of the diet.

Management Phase Guidelines

The Management Phase is similar in many ways to the previous phases in our plan. You're still eating four meals a day, spaced roughly four hours apart. Include at least two of the 20/20 Foods with each meal, one of which can be hot or cold green tea. Besides the Management Phase meal options we'll discuss below, all of the meals in Phases 2 and 3 are open to you. Just don't select Phase 1 meals during the Management Phase—those were designed specifically for the initial part of this plan. You are no longer in that phase.

The Hunger and Fullness Scale is still your valuable ally in this campaign. Use it to determine when you are full, which should now always be your prompt to put down the fork. Sensible splurges are most definitely allowed during the Management Phase, as long as you follow the rules we laid down in chapter 8. If old habits start to creep back in and you find yourself eating for the wrong reasons, remember to take those essential 30 seconds before each meal and assign positive value to the food you are about to enjoy.

Management Phase Meal Planning

Planning your Management Phase meals is easy.

Here's how: First, select two 20/20 Foods that you would like to eat. Then, see where the foods you selected fit within the meal framework below and fill in your choices. *Note:* Mustard and green tea are great choices, but they don't fill any of the blanks. If you're not sure where the 20/20 Foods for your meal fit, refer to the list below that breaks them down by category.

Power Protein = _____

Prime Produce = _____

Super Starch = _____

Fit Fat = _____

Power Proteins:
Whey protein

Tofu

Chickpeas

Lentils

Yogurt (nonfat)

Eggs

Cod

Prime Produce:
Apples

Dried plums (prunes)

Raisins

Greens (any kind of leafy greens)

Super Starch:
Rye

Other:
Green tea

Mustard

Fit Fats:
Coconut oil

Pistachios (roasted, unsalted)

Olive oil

Almonds

Walnuts

Peanut butter (natural)

Round out your meal by selecting other foods of your choice from the lists in appendix C to fill in the remaining blanks. Each list begins with the correct portions for each category of food. Every meal should include the following mix:

- 1 Power Protein
- 1–2 Prime Produce
- 1 Super Starch
- 1 Fit Fat

Here's an example of how to use this formula.

1. My two 20/20 Foods choices are spinach and lentils.
   Fill in where they fit:

   Power Protein = Lentils

   Prime Produce = Spinach

   Super Starch = _____

   Fit Fat = _____

2. Round out meal by filling in blanks and portions:

   1 Power Protein = 1/2 cup lentils

   1–2 Prime Produce = 2 cups spinach, 1 tomato

   1 Super Starch = 1/2 cup fingerling potatoes

   1 Fit Fat = 1/4 ripe avocado

Men: Don't forget to double the portions of each food in one of the daily meals you consume, prior to your most active time of day. If a food you like is not on the lists, enjoy it as your sensible splurge.

As always, use the Hunger and Fullness Scale to determine when to stop eating.

Note: You can find a complete list of common power proteins, prime produce, super starches, and fit fats in appendix C.

Sample Meals

On the following pages are some sample meals to get you started, but I encourage you to get creative. You should not feel like these are the *only* meals you can eat! That would get pretty boring. The whole idea is to keep up with plenty of variety and have fun seasoning and flavoring your food, because this time you are not rebelling or feeling like you're in a prison of bland, flavorless foods. (* = 20/20 Food)

Breakfast

PLUM PISTACHIO OATMEAL

Slice or chop 1/4 cup dried plums*; set aside. Combine 1/4 cup unsweetened whey protein powder* with 1/4 cup dry rolled oats, add hot water, and stir. Top with the dried plums and 2 tablespoons pistachios.

APPLE WALNUT CEREAL

Chop 1 small apple* and mix with a 6-ounce cup of nonfat (0%) vanilla Greek yogurt,* along with 1/2 cup unsweetened spoon-sized shredded wheat cereal and 2 tablespoons unsalted raw or dry-roasted walnuts,* or layer the ingredients parfait-style.

OPEN-FACED EGG AVOCADO SANDWICH

Cook 1 large egg* any way you'd like (sunny-side up, scrambled, or hard boiled). Toast 1 slice whole-grain rye bread,* spread with 1/4 of a ripe avocado, and top with the egg. Serve with a side dish of 1 cup cubed melon.

Blueberry Parfait

Layer a 6-ounce cup of nonfat (0%) vanilla Greek yogurt parfait-style with 1 cup blueberries, 1/4 cup rye flakes,* and 2 tablespoons almonds.* (Option: toast the rye flakes in a toaster oven or on a cookie sheet in the oven.)

Peanut Butter Banana Crackers

Spread 1 tablespoon natural peanut butter* on 2 rye crisps.* Top with 1/2 sliced banana and pair with 1 cup chilled skim milk.

Pistachio Cottage Cheese Spread

Spread 2 rye crisps* with 1/2 cup low-fat cottage cheese and top with 2 tablespoons pistachios.* Serve with 1 cup of grapes as a side dish.

Open-Faced Tofu Sandwich

Sauté 1 cup spinach* in 2 teaspoons extra-virgin olive oil* with seasonings of your choice, such as minced garlic and Italian herbs. Toast 1 slice whole-grain bread, top with the cooked spinach, then add 1/5 of a 14-ounce package of chilled, sliced tofu.* (Option: crumble the tofu and sauté with the spinach.)

Lunch

Chilled Lentil and Wild Rice Salad

Place 1 cup romaine lettuce* in a salad bowl. Top with 1/2 cup cooked lentils* and 1/3 cup cooked, chilled wild rice. Drizzle with 2 teaspoons extra-virgin olive oil* and, if desired, season with a squeeze of fresh lemon, minced garlic, and cracked black pepper.

OPEN-FACED TUNA SANDWICH

Chop 1 cup arugula* and mix into 3 ounces chunk light tuna (canned in water) along with 2 tablespoons sunflower seeds. If desired, season with a tablespoon of balsamic vinegar and Italian herbs. Spoon the tuna mixture onto 1 slice whole-grain rye bread,* toasted or untoasted.

CHICKPEA AND VEGGIE PASTA SALAD

Toss 1/2 cup chickpeas* with 1 cup sliced grape tomatoes, red onion, and mushrooms; 1/3 cup cooked, chilled whole-grain penne; and 2 teaspoons extra-virgin olive oil.* If desired, season with minced garlic and herbs of your choice, such as fresh or dried basil.

TOFU, CORN, AND AVOCADO SALAD

Crumble 1/5 of a 14-ounce package tofu* or slice into cubes. Place 1 cup mixed greens* in a salad bowl. Top with tofu, 1/3 cup corn, and 1/4 of a ripe avocado. (Option: roast corn on a cookie sheet in the oven, and season salad with herbs of your choice, such as fresh or dried cilantro.)

SALMON AND WALNUT LETTUCE WRAPS

Crumble or crush 2 rye crisps* and chop or crumble 3 ounces salmon; set aside. Fill 3 outer romaine lettuce leaves* with salmon, top with 1/2 cup chopped tomatoes and red onion, then sprinkle with rye crisps and 2 tablespoons unsalted raw or dry-roasted walnuts.* If desired, lightly drizzle with balsamic vinegar and/or a squeeze of fresh lemon.

Black Bean and Rice Platter

Sauté 1 cup red bell peppers, onions, and spinach* in 2 teaspoons extra-virgin olive oil.* If desired, season with minced garlic and chipotle seasoning. Serve with side dishes of 1/2 cup cooked black beans and 1/3 cup cooked brown rice.

Citrus Chicken Salad

Chop or mince 3 ounces cooked boneless, skinless chicken breast; set aside. Place 1 cup mixed greens* in a salad bowl. Top with sections from 1 small tangerine, then 1/3 cup cooked, chilled brown rice, and sprinkle with 2 tablespoons almonds.* If desired, season with herbs of your choice, such as thyme.

Snacks

Apple Walnut Muesli

Chop 1 small apple* and mix with a 6-ounce cup of nonfat (0%) vanilla Greek yogurt,* along with 1/4 cup dry raw or toasted rolled oats and 2 tablespoons unsalted raw or dry-roasted walnuts,* or layer the ingredients parfait-style. If desired, add a dash of cinnamon or apple pie spice. (Option: toast the oats in a toaster oven or on a cookie sheet in the oven.)

Roasted Chickpeas and Fresh Veggies

Toss 1/2 cup chickpeas* in 2 teaspoons extra-virgin olive oil* and roast in the oven on a cookie sheet or in foil until golden. Serve with 1 cup raw baby carrots and grape tomatoes and 2 rye crisps.*

Egg and Avocado Snack

Spread 2 rye crisps* with 1/4 of a ripe avocado and top with 1 large, sliced hard-boiled egg.* Pair with 1 cup pink grapefruit sections.

CHERRY SMOOTHIE AND PEANUT BUTTER CRACKERS

In a blender, combine a 6-ounce cup of nonfat (0%) vanilla Greek yogurt,* 1/4 cup unsweetened whey protein powder,* and 3/4 cup frozen pitted cherries (add water to thin mixture if desired). Spread 2 rye crisps* with 1 tablespoon natural peanut butter* and pair with smoothie.

FRUIT, CHEESE, AND CRISPS

Enjoy 1 reduced-fat string cheese, 1 small pear, 2 rye crisps,* and 2 tablespoons unsalted raw or dry-roasted walnuts* individually or, if desired, slice pear and serve on top of crackers.

PLUM COTTAGE CHEESE CRUNCH

Finely chop 1/4 cup dried plums* and fold into 1/2 cup low-fat cottage cheese along with 2 tablespoons sunflower seeds.* Spread mixture onto 2 rye crisps.*

FETA CHEESE AND PESTO CRACKERS

Spread 2 teaspoons pesto onto 2 rye crisps.* Top with 1/4 cup crumbled feta cheese and enjoy with 1 small apple* cut into wedges.

Dinner

CHICKEN, SAUTÉED SPINACH, AND CORN

Sauté 1 cup spinach* and 1/2 cup corn in 2 teaspoons extra-virgin olive oil.* If desired, add minced garlic and herbs of your choice, such as cilantro and/or crushed red pepper. Serve with 3 ounces cooked boneless, skinless chicken breast.

Salmon Dinner Salad

Cube 1/2 cup skin-on red potatoes and roast in the oven until golden. Place 1 cup fresh spinach* in a salad bowl. Top with 3 ounces cooked salmon, then the potatoes, and sprinkle with 2 tablespoons almonds.* If desired, lightly drizzle with balsamic vinegar, add a squeeze of fresh lemon, and dust with cracked black pepper.

Shrimp and Spinach Stir-Fry

Stir-fry 1 cup spinach* and onions along with 3 ounces shrimp in 2 teaspoons coconut oil.* If desired, add seasonings like fresh ginger, minced garlic, and crushed red pepper. Serve over 1/3 cup brown rice.

Roasted Turkey, Kale, and Potatoes

Roast 1/2 cup fingerling potatoes and 3 ounces roasted skinless, boneless turkey breast in the oven until cooked through. Sauté 1 cup chopped kale* in 2 teaspoons extra-virgin olive oil.* If desired, add minced garlic, a squeeze of fresh lemon juice, and cracked black pepper.

Lentil and Wild Rice Sauté

Sauté 1 cup cauliflower, carrots, asparagus, and onions along with 1/2 cup cooked lentils* in 2 teaspoons extra-virgin olive oil.* If desired, add minced garlic and Italian herbs. Serve over 1/3 cup wild rice.

Baked Cod, Veggies, and Wild Rice

Sauté 1 cup eggplant, tomatoes, onions, and mushrooms in 2 teaspoons extra-virgin olive oil.* If desired, add minced garlic and Italian herbs. Serve with 1/3 cup wild rice and 3 ounces baked cod.*

> ### Coconut Chicken and Spinach Pasta
>
> Cut 3 ounces roasted skinless, boneless chicken breast into cubes. Sauté 1 cup spinach* in 2 teaspoons coconut oil* and mix with cubed chicken and 1/3 cup cooked whole-grain penne. If desired, season with minced garlic and cracked black pepper.

Pitfalls to Weight Management

Remember those pitfalls I briefly mentioned earlier in this chapter? Well, here they are, and here's what you can do to avoid them.

Self-Sabotage Masquerading as Celebration: The first pitfall to avoid has to do with how you react to the excitement of reaching your goal. Go back and review the healthy rewards you wrote down in chapter 8, and make sure you are rewarding yourself for this achievement in a nonfood, healthy and positive manner. In other words, don't sabotage yourself and your weight loss by running out to eat, drink, and be merry until you're busting at the seams! You can experience the same euphoric payoff of a celebration without bingeing on food or alcohol. This is true going forward too—anytime you're seeking a reward (e.g., after a long day of work, a promotion, or just a fun weekend), make sure you're not actually punishing yourself.

"Fixed Fat" Beliefs: Once you've lost a significant amount of weight, other people might take notice and pay you compliments. If you hear what they're saying, but every time you look in the mirror you still see a fat person staring back at you, it could be that you've got some "fixed fat" beliefs about yourself.

These beliefs are dangerous because they limit you psychologically and keep you from accepting your own success. They can ultimately set you up for gaining the weight back. Combat these beliefs by getting comfortable looking in the mirror and getting used to your new appearance, forcing yourself to do things that once made you uneasy (such as wearing a bathing suit or attending parties you'd usually skip), and exercising even more to improve your body image. The goal is to

Guilt Gets You Nowhere

In this plan, I'm not asking you to strive for perfection—I'm asking you to strive for excellence. You are going to be less than perfect, and that's OK because what we're looking for is a pattern across time. It's not what you do on any given day; it's what you do on *most* days. There's nothing you can do today to lose all of the weight, and there's nothing you can do today to keep you from losing all of it. So if you deviate, or maybe inadvertently eat something that you thought was healthy but turned out to be loaded with sugar, for example, it's not the end of the world. You'll bounce back.

But if you mess up and then let yourself feel consumed with guilt over it, you'll endanger your success. As we say in Texas, guilt is like rocking in a rocking chair—it's something to do, but it doesn't get you anywhere. You don't need guilt on this diet, because this diet is driven by programming, not emotion. So, if you skip a workout or eat a doughnut one day, do not fall into the guilt trap and risk returning to the same emotion-fueled behavior that got you here. Get up, dust yourself off, and carry on. Remember how getting off track makes you feel so that you don't repeat the behavior tomorrow.

replace any self-defeating thoughts with positive, realistic affirmations and alternatives.

Remember when you came up with your 20/20 vision of the future? Well, that future is now your present if you've reached your weight loss goals or you're getting close. So what's stopping you from appreciating the vision you know you deserve and have worked so hard to achieve?

Failure to Self-Monitor: You need to stay in the habit of keeping tabs on your weight and measurements to make sure you're remaining within a healthy range. Monitor yourself regularly to ensure that you're still applying positive meaning to your meals, following the sensible splurge rules, and maintaining your no-fail environments. Don't relax your efforts so much that you lose sight of your goals and let your weight creep back up.

Acute Stress or Crisis: You can't predict when life will throw you a curveball, but you can decide now that when tragedy strikes or something triggers an acute stress response, you will still put yourself and your goals first by not allowing emotions to drastically change your eating and exercise behavior. We've talked about how you will no longer use food to solve any problems other than genuine hunger, so when stressful times hit, that's no time to let go of that pact you've made with yourself. That may have been your old way of coping, but that doesn't work for the new you. You know it doesn't help the situation. In fact, it will probably make it worse. Talk about this with one or several of your supporters now so that they can remind you and help strengthen you when the time comes.

Stealthy Saboteurs: Continue to keep your guard up against saboteurs. They sometimes seem to come out of the woodwork, and you might be surprised how vicious even a close friend can be when they're overcome with jealousy. Your success makes them feel like more of a failure. Beware of friends or family members who try to get you off track. You know what's right for you. If they're pushing cake, pizza, or ice cream in your direction, politely decline. Turn to your supporters, and don't let the stealthy saboteurs get under your skin.

Are You Stressed from Overscheduling?

Especially if you're a parent, it can be very easy to fall into the trap of overscheduling and spreading yourself too thin. If you hit the ground running every morning and feel like you can't take a breath until bedtime, you could be putting your weight management in jeopardy. If you don't put yourself first, you could very easily fall back into the old habits that made you gain the weight in the first place. Use these tips to get your hectic life back under control:

Examine Your Motivation: Are you trying to be all things to all people, often playing the role of "hero" or "martyr"? Make sure your motivations are healthy ones that allow you to take care of yourself first and foremost so you can be there fully for others.

Get OK with Delegating: The old adage "if you want it done right, do it yourself" just doesn't work across the board. You've got to conserve your time and energy by delegating tasks to others. And if your husband doesn't fold the laundry as perfectly as you do, is that really going to matter in the grand scheme of things?

"No" Is Not a Bad Word: Identify the responsibilities you've taken on, and if any of them can go by the wayside to create more time in your schedule, then they need to go. And when new demands on your time arise, don't be afraid to politely say, "I have enough on my plate right now, so I'm going to pass on this opportunity." If you keep giving of yourself and never saying "no," others will continue to take from you. Refusing to jeopardize your personal goals in exchange for doing everything asked of you does not make you a bad person.

Schedule "Me" Time: If you can't remember the last time you spent an hour doing something *you* want to do, then you need to pull out the calendar and schedule time that is yours and yours alone. This needs to become a part of your weekly routine in order to maintain your mental, physical, and emotional health.

You now have the tools you need to create and enjoy meals, whether at home or at a restaurant, that will support your weight loss goals. You also have a three-phase plan that you can repeat until you have achieved your ideal, healthy weight, and a management system that will help you sustain this weight for the rest of your life.

In the next chapter, I'm going to show you some of the incredible ways that the inner workings of your body can be transformed by losing weight in this healthy manner. I hope it will open your eyes to the power you have to change your destiny with the adjustments you are making to your lifestyle. The future is not yet written, and the pen is in your hand. By making the bold decision to change the way you treat your body, you are writing a new, healthier, and longer future for your life.

13

YOUR RETURN
TO HEALTH

What lies behind you and what lies in front of you,
pales in comparison to what lies inside of you.
—Ralph Waldo Emerson

Riddle: What's the world's most dangerous weapon? Answer: the fork.

It's true! The fork destroys more lives, creates more disease, and takes more years off people's lives than all the typical weapons you might be picturing combined. Eating the wrong foods can seriously endanger your health, but the opposite is also true—eating the *right* foods, the ones we've been talking about, can improve your health.

I want to talk to you about all the ways in which losing weight on this plan can protect and preserve your health.

In chapter 4, I asked you to think about all of the ways your weight has been standing in the way of what you want. In our survey, we asked about people's motivation for losing weight, and found that 48.6%—just about half of the respondents—rated "health concerns" as a 10 out of 10. It was their *top* motivation for wanting to lose weight. Another question in the survey asked whether a medical doctor had recommended that they lose weight, to which 62.7 percent answered "yes." Now, that's serious.

On some level, you know your health has been jeopardized by your weight problem. But I want to offer you hope by showing you that you can help improve your health through healthy eating and exercise.

Do You Have a High-Mileage Heart?

The average person's heart pumps blood through 60,000 miles of blood vessels every single day. Yes, you read that right! Since your heart is working as much as 30 percent harder to pump blood throughout your body if you're significantly overweight, you can just tack on an extra 18,000 miles of blood vessels through which your heart is pumping blood per 24-hour period.

Think of it this way: it's 24,000 miles around the entire Earth, so if you're overweight, your heart is pumping blood the equivalent of three-quarters of the way around the whole planet every single *day*. You're asking a lot of your heart. But reaching a healthy weight through eating right and exercise can help your health, including the health of your heart.

Health Changes

Let's look together at some of the positive health changes that scientists have attributed to weight loss. A healthy diet and exercise can help make you healthier overall, though any specific changes to your health are based on complex factors, such as your genetics. I wanted you to be aware of potential positive health changes to help motivate you to take charge of your health, but you should discuss any specific health concerns with your doctor to determine the best plan of action for you.

1. Smaller Waistline: In the survey, I asked a question about which body part you most want to change. A whopping 93.7 percent of people chose "belly." No one likes having extra jiggle around their midsection, but there are clear-cut reasons why belly fat endangers your health. That fat beneath your abdominal wall can increase inflammation throughout your body, raise your blood pressure, slow your metabolism, and lower your immunity.

2. Lower Resting Heart Rate: Your heart is a pump. At its most basic level, it is a pump whose job it is to circulate blood throughout your body. Your resting heart rate is the number of times your heart beats per minute while you're at complete rest. This is an important indication of your heart's health because if it's working overtime even when you're sitting around, you can imagine how hard it's pumping when you're active and moving. If you're overweight or obese, your heart rate may be higher than average. Losing weight through healthy diet and exercise may help you lower your heart rate.

3. Breathing Easier: If you've felt out of breath going up one flight of stairs or you've had to take a break just walking to your car from the grocery store, then you know the effects that your weight and physical fitness have on your lungs. But as you lose the weight and get in shape, you may notice that you are able to breathe a little easier and do not get as fatigued by everyday physical tasks.

4. Sharper Mind: Junk food and fast food have been shown in studies to impair brain function. Think about that for a second: the food you eat has a direct impact on how your brain works. Eating healthier could not only affect your weight but may help you to feel less "foggy" and to think more clearly.

5. More Energy: Eating healthy and exercising could also help you feel more energetic. Carrying around extra weight could be one of the reasons you feel worn out. For example, if you are 20 pounds overweight, just imagine picking up a 20-pound piece of furniture, strapping it to your back, and hauling it around everywhere you go. That's basically what you've been doing with the extra weight. So as you lose weight, you might find the get-up-and-go that you've been missing all this time.

6. Better Sleep: Studies suggest that people who eat healthy are more likely to sleep better. Regular exercise is also an important factor in helping you rest easier.

7. Blood Pressure: Lowering your sodium intake and adding plenty of whole fruits and vegetables to your diet may help you maintain a healthy blood pressure. Exercise can also have an effect on your blood pressure.

8. Cholesterol: Healthy eating and exercise can also be an important part of maintaining a healthy cholesterol.

9. C-Reactive Protein: This test is an indication of how much inflammation there is in your body. Doctors now believe that inflammation is at the core of most modern-day diseases, including heart disease, diabetes, cancer, and more. A healthy, balanced diet and exercise could have an effect on your C-reactive protein level.

10. Blood Sugars: Bad food habits such as large portions, erratic meal schedules, and high-fat, high-sugar, low-fiber foods can all wreak havoc on your blood sugar. Like other effects on health, healthy eating and exercise can help support your blood glucose levels and help your body process sugar and insulin.

Acknowledge and Attribute

In chapter 3, we talked about observing yourself succeeding at something, acknowledging that you are living to your potential, and making a positive attribution to yourself regarding that competency. Right now, I want you to observe and acknowledge that you are doing something good for your health by committing to losing weight.

Think about any health-related changes you have experienced since starting this diet, such an overall sense of feeling better. Write it down, and then recognize that you are someone who has made their health a priority.

What's Age Got to Do with It?

Ask any woman over the age of 40 if it's harder to lose weight (and easier to gain it) and you will hear a resounding YES! It's an unfortunate fact of life that aging, and specifically the fluctuations in hormones associated with aging, has a drastic effect on weight, particularly in women.

Yes, changing hormones make women's bodies more likely to store fat and harder for them to lose it. If you're "of a certain age" and carrying around a lot of extra weight, you should be aware that research shows you're at an even *higher* risk of type 2 diabetes, various cancers (including colorectal and breast cancer), and heart disease than when you were younger.

So just like with weight loss resistance that I discussed in chapter 11, if you are older and worried about being able to lose weight, I recommend that you talk to your doctor about the best course of action.

Even though it might not be as easy to drop 10 pounds as it was when you were 20 years old, with the help of your doctor, you *can* do it.

But What if Fat Is in My Genes?

As scientists continue to discover more about the human genome, they're finding out that we have genetic predispositions for numerous health risks, and obesity is no exception. Lately, there has been some buzz in the media about something referred to as the "fat gene," or "obesity gene." It's actually an extremely common genetic variant, which more than a third of the American population carries. But our genes are not the sole determinants of our destiny. Far from it!

Even if you carry this gene variant, and even if you are overweight or obese, there were a lot of other factors that had to exist in order for you to get that way. Your environment and your decisions about food, exercise, and lifestyle, also likely played a role at how you arrived at this point. Your genetics may have given your body the green light, but ultimately, *you* were driving that car.

But, studies suggest that healthy eating and exercise can play an important role in helping you reach and maintain a healthy weight. In one meta-analysis of 45 studies on over 200,000 adults, researchers found that of people who have the obesity gene, those who were getting even a little physical exercise were at a 27 percent lower risk of being overweight or obese. That's all very encouraging!

So you see, your genes do not control you. Even your DNA shouldn't stand in your way of a healthier, happier life.

Returning to health means being able to live your life to its fullest potential now and in the future. So take control over your health now and start implementing this plan. I don't want you to miss out on all the incredible things life has to offer, and all that *you* have to offer the world, because you were too scared to make a change.

Don't you wonder what amazing things you could accomplish if you turned the tide on your life, lost weight, and allowed your body systems to function at a higher level? Stop wondering and start transforming. It could be the best decision you'll ever make.

14

CONCLUSION:
THE NEW YOU

I believe we can create moments in time in which all things wrong can be made right. In this book, I've told you what you have to be willing to do in order to succeed at righting the wrongs when it comes to your weight, your health, and your self-image, and hopefully, you've already started doing those things every day.

In a book I wrote called *Life Code*, I included a playbook of important strategies, mindsets, tactics, and behaviors to create more of what you want in your life, which I referred to as the "Sweet 16." The very first strategy is: you must have a defined "image" and never go out of character.

Since you've begun losing weight and resetting your health, how has your defined image changed? Are you projecting a persona of good fitness because your coworkers and friends see you going to the gym on a regular basis? Do others perceive you as someone who makes nutritious, healthful food choices because of the way you order when you're at a restaurant? Does your family now understand that your health is a top priority because you create time for yourself in the schedule?

I'm betting your defined image has shifted in more ways than you might realize, so now you need to embrace that. Identify your new-found strengths and commit to the healthy image and statement that you're projecting.

You do what works for you in your life. The difference between now and before you started this diet is that you're seeking a different end goal. Before, you ate what you ate, thought what you thought, and did what you did because that worked to generate the same results they had always generated. That was enough for you then, but it's not enough for you anymore. Now, you've set your sights on a new weight and way of life, so you're doing what works to generate those *new* end goals. But it doesn't mean you're immune to backsliding, so if you feel yourself giving up some of your control over your habits and behaviors, return to the pages of this book and the phases of this diet to regain your command.

Another important strategy from *Life Code* is to master the system (be it your workplace, your relationships—anything) and figure out a way to make it work for you. The better you know the system, the better you understand the game and how it's played, thus, the more likely you are to win. This is true of this diet. Learn it, understand it, and make the lifestyle changes necessary to implement it so you can win at losing weight now and keep winning in the long run.

I want you to get what you want, and then *keep* it and build on it. By finally losing the weight that was holding you back and doing it in a healthy manner, you've opened the door to brand new opportunities to live your life, your way. You've fundamentally changed your view of yourself and how you approach everything. Now, you've seen yourself start a diet with habits that last a lifetime, and you can look forward to a lot of *first* times of new, healthy, positive experiences ahead.

Here's to the new you!

APPENDIX A

Grocery Lists

Phase 1 Shopping List (* = 20/20 Food)

DAIRY

Eggs, large*

Yogurt—nonfat (0%) vanilla Greek yogurts (made with real sugar, not artificial sweetener)*

FRESH FRUIT

Apples, small (about 2 ¾″), your choice (Red Delicious, Golden Delicious, Granny Smith, etc.)*

Lemons

Plums, dried*

Raisins*

FRESH VEGGIES/PRODUCE

Chickpeas, bagged or canned*

Garlic

Lentils, bagged, steamed vacuum sealed, or canned*

Tofu, extra firm*

Mixed greens, your choice (arugula, baby mixed greens, bok choy, endive, field greens, radicchio, red leaf lettuce, romaine, baby spinach, watercress, etc.)*

SPICES AND OILS

Cinnamon

Dijon mustard*

Coconut oil*

Olive oil, extra virgin*

NUTS

Almonds, unsalted raw or dry roasted*

Peanut butter, all natural*

Pistachios, unsalted, shelled*

Walnuts, halved*

PASTAS, OATS, AND GRAINS

Rye crisps, whole grain

MEATS/PROTEINS

Cod, fresh*

Whey protein powder, unsweetened*

BEVERAGES

Natural green tea*

Phase 2 Shopping List (* = 20/20 Food)

Keep in mind: This grocery list covers everything in all of the Phase 2 meals. If there are certain meals you don't plan to make, you don't need to purchase all the ingredients.

DAIRY

Eggs, large*

Yogurt—nonfat (0%) vanilla Greek yogurts (made with real sugar, not artificial sweetener)*

FRESH FRUIT

Apples, small (about 2 ¾"), your choice (Red Delicious, Golden Delicious, Granny Smith, etc.)*

Blueberries

Grapes, seedless, your choice (red, green, black)

Lemons

Oranges

Plums, dried*

Raisins*

FRESH VEGGIES/PRODUCE

Avocado

Carrots

Chickpeas, bagged or canned*

Cilantro

Garlic

Grape tomatoes

Lentils, bagged, steamed vacuum sealed, or canned*

Romaine leaves*

Mixed greens, your choice (arugula, baby mixed greens, bok choy, endive, field greens, radicchio, red leaf lettuce, romaine, baby spinach, watercress, etc.)*

Mushrooms

Spinach*

Tofu, extra firm*

Tomatoes

FROZEN FRUIT AND VEGGIES
Blueberries, unsweetened

Corn

SPICES AND OILS
Balsamic vinegar

Black pepper

Cayenne pepper (optional)

Cinnamon

Coconut oil*

Crushed red pepper (optional)

Dijon mustard*

Dill, dried

Italian herb seasoning, salt free, dried

Olive oil, extra virgin*

Vegetable broth, low sodium

NUTS
Almonds, unsalted raw or dry roasted*

Cashews

Peanut butter, all natural*

Pistachios, unsalted, shelled*

Sunflower seeds

Walnuts, halved*

PASTAS, OATS, AND GRAINS
Brown rice

Oats, rolled

Rye bread, whole grain*

Rye crisps, whole grain

Rye pasta, whole grain*

MEATS/PROTEINS
Black beans, bagged or low-sodium canned

Chicken breast, boneless, skinless

Cod, fresh*

Tuna, chunk light, canned in water

Whey protein powder, unsweetened*

BEVERAGES
Natural green tea*

Phase 3 Shopping List (* = 20/20 Food)

Phase 3 includes a much wider variety of foods, and the recipes don't share as many ingredients as Phases 1 and 2. If you know there are certain meals you like that require specific ingredients, focus on those rather than buying everything on the list and overflowing your kitchen.

DAIRY

Cottage cheese, low fat

Eggs, large*

Mini round cheeses (roughly 70 calories each)

Skim milk

Yogurt—nonfat (0%) vanilla Greek yogurts (made with real sugar, not artificial sweetener)*

FRESH FRUIT

Apples, small (about 2 ¾″), your choice (Red Delicious, Golden Delicious, Granny Smith, etc.)*

Bananas

Blueberries

Cherries, unsweetened, pitted

Grapes, seedless, your choice (red, green, black)

Kiwis

Lemons

Limes

Oranges

Peaches, medium

Pears, small, your choice (Anjou, Bartlett, Bosc, Comice, etc.)

Plums, dried*

Raisins*

Raspberries

Strawberries

Tangerines

FRESH VEGGIES/PRODUCE

Avocado

Basil leaves

Bell peppers, green

Bell peppers, red

Broccoli

Carrots

Cauliflower

Chickpeas, bagged or canned*

Cilantro

Eggplant

Garlic

Ginger

Grape tomatoes

Green beans

Lentils, bagged, steamed vacuum sealed, or canned*

FRESH VEGGIES/PRODUCE (*continued*)

Mixed greens, your choice
  (arugula, baby mixed greens,
  bok choy, endive, field greens,
  radicchio, red leaf lettuce,
  romaine, baby spinach,
  watercress, etc.)*

Mushrooms

Onion

Parsley

Potatoes, Red Bliss

Red onion

Romaine leaves*

Spaghetti squash

Spinach*

Sundried tomatoes

Tofu, extra firm*

Tomatoes

Zucchini

FROZEN FRUITS AND VEGGIES

Blueberries, unsweetened

Mango, unsweetened

Peaches, unsweetened

Pineapple, unsweetened

Strawberries, unsweetened

Corn

SPICES AND OILS

Balsamic vinegar

Black pepper

Cayenne pepper (optional)

Cinnamon

Cloves

Coconut oil*

Crushed red pepper

Dijon mustard*

Dill, dried

Garlic powder (not garlic salt)

Italian herb seasoning, salt free,
  dried

Olive oil, extra virgin*

Parsley, dried

Vegetable broth, low sodium

NUTS

Almonds, unsalted raw or dry
  roasted*

Cashews

Peanut butter, all natural*

Pistachios, unsalted, shelled*

Sunflower seeds

Walnuts, halved*

PASTAS, OATS, AND GRAINS

Brown rice

Corn tortillas, whole grain

Couscous, whole wheat

Oats, rolled

Penne, whole grain

Pita, whole grain

Quinoa

Rye bread, whole grain*

PASTAS, OATS, AND GRAINS (*continued*)

Rye crisps, whole grain

Rye flakes, whole grain*

Rye pasta, whole grain*

Shredded wheat cereal, unsweetened, spoon sized

Soba noodles

Wild rice

MEATS/PROTEINS

Black beans, bagged or low-sodium canned

Cannellini beans

Chicken breast, boneless, skinless

Cod, fresh*

Salmon, fresh

Turkey, ground, extra lean

Shrimp, medium, peeled, deveined (frozen, thawed is OK)

Tuna, chunk light, canned in water

Turkey breast, oven roasted, boneless, skinless

Whey protein powder, unsweetened*

OTHER

Olives, Mediterranean or Greek, your choice (green, black, Kalamata)

Pesto, jarred

BEVERAGES

Natural green tea*

APPENDIX B

Phase 3 Meals: The 20-Day Attain

Breakfast Options

APPLE ALMOND CEREAL

Chop 2 tablespoons almonds; set aside. Pour 1 cup skim milk over 1/2 cup unsweetened spoon-sized shredded wheat cereal and garnish with a dash of cinnamon. Top with 1 small chopped apple of your choice, skin on. Top with almonds.

PLUM PEANUT BUTTER OATMEAL

In a small bowl, mix together 1/4 cup each unsweetened whey protein powder and rolled oats. Pour hot water over the mixture until you reach desired consistency (suggested amount: 1/4 cup water). Swirl in 2 teaspoons all-natural peanut butter and garnish with a dash of cinnamon and 5 chopped dried plums.

STRAWBERRY PLUM WALNUT CEREAL

Chop 2 tablespoons walnuts and 2 dried plums; set aside. Pour 1 cup skim milk over 1/2 cup unsweetened spoon-sized shredded wheat cereal and garnish with a dash of cinnamon. Top with 1/2 cup sliced strawberries and the chopped plums and walnuts.

Open-Faced Tofu Dijon Sandwich

In a small bowl, whisk 2 teaspoons Dijon mustard with 1 teaspoon water, 1 teaspoon lemon juice, 2 teaspoons extra-virgin olive oil, and 1/2 teaspoon minced garlic. Coat sliced extra-firm tofu (1/5 of a 14-ounce package) with mustard sauce. Place 1/2 cup spinach on top of 1 slice (1 ounce) whole-grain rye bread (fresh or toasted). Top with tofu and enjoy with 1 small apple of your choice, skin on.

Veggie Scramble over Brown Rice

Whisk 1 large egg and season with 1/4 teaspoon minced garlic, 1 teaspoon fresh or 1/2 teaspoon dried parsley, and 1/16 teaspoon ground black pepper. In a medium pan, scramble the egg with 1 tablespoon extra-virgin olive oil, 1/4 cup diced tomato, 2 tablespoons minced onion, and 1 cup fresh spinach. Serve over 1/2 cup cooked brown rice (fluffy, not packed).

Apple Pistachio French Toast

Chop 1 small apple of your choice, skin on, and sauté in a small pan in 1 teaspoon coconut oil until tender; set aside. In a medium bowl, beat 1 large egg. Soak 1 slice (1 ounce) whole-grain rye bread in the egg. Transfer to sauté pan (pour any excess egg over bread) and cook until each side is golden brown. Top with sautéed apple and garnish with 1 tablespoon unsalted shelled pistachios, chopped. (Option: leave pistachios whole.)

Peach Coconut Smoothie

In a blender, combine a single-serve container of nonfat (0%) vanilla Greek yogurt, 1/4 cup unsweetened whey protein powder, 3/4 cup frozen unsweetened peaches, and 1/4 cup water. Whip until smooth. Add 1/2 tablespoon coconut oil, 1 tablespoon rolled oats, and a handful of ice, and whip to desired consistency.

Peanut Butter Blueberry Toast

In a small bowl, sprinkle 1 cup fresh blueberries with a dash of cinnamon and mash slightly; set aside. Spread 1 slice (1 ounce) whole-grain bread with 1 tablespoon all-natural peanut butter. Top with mashed berries. Pair with a single-serve container of nonfat (0%) vanilla Greek yogurt. (Option: use 3/4 cup frozen, thawed blueberries in place of fresh.)

Plum Walnut Cottage Cheese Toast

Chop 2 tablespoons walnuts and 5 dried plums; set aside. Spread 1 slice (1 ounce) whole-grain bread with 1/2 cup low-fat cottage cheese and garnish with a dash of cinnamon. Top with plums and walnuts.

Spinach Omelet with Avocado Toast

Whisk 1 large egg and season with 1/4 teaspoon minced garlic. In a medium pan, cook the egg with 1 cup fresh spinach. Pair with 1 slice (1 ounce) whole-grain rye bread spread with 1/4 of a ripe avocado. Pair with 3/4 cup seedless grapes.

Pistachio Cherry Oatmeal

Chop or crush 2 tablespoons unsalted shelled pistachios; set aside. Place 1 cup frozen cherries in a small saucepan with 2 tablespoons water and a dash of cloves. Stir over medium heat until cherries are soft and water has evaporated. In a small bowl, mix together 1/4 cup each unsweetened whey protein powder and rolled oats. Pour hot water over the mixture until you reach desired consistency (suggested amount: 1/4 cup water). Top with cherries and garnish with pistachios. (Option: warm cherries in microwave, mash slightly, and season with a dash of cloves.)

Kiwi Almond Parfait

Chop 2 tablespoons unsalted raw or dry-roasted almonds; set aside. Layer a single-serve container of nonfat (0%) vanilla Greek yogurt with 2 chopped small kiwis, 2 tablespoons rolled oats, and the chopped almonds. (Option: toast the rolled oats in a toaster oven or in a conventional oven on a cookie sheet until they are crispy.)

Mango Coconut Smoothie

In a blender, combine a single-serve container of nonfat (0%) vanilla Greek yogurt, 1/4 cup unsweetened whey protein powder, 3/4 cup frozen unsweetened mango, and 1/4 cup water. Whip until smooth. Add 1/2 tablespoon coconut oil, 1 tablespoon rolled oats, and a handful of ice, and whip to desired consistency.

Peanut Butter Banana Toast

Spread 1 slice (1 ounce) toasted whole-grain bread with 1 table-spoon all-natural peanut butter. Top with 1/2 cup sliced banana and a dash of cinnamon. Pair with a single-serve container of non-fat (0%) vanilla Greek yogurt.

Pear Walnut Parfait

Toast 2 tablespoons whole-grain rye flakes in a toaster oven or on a cookie sheet in a 350°F preheated oven for 5 minutes or until they look slightly browned and have a nutty aroma. Chop a small pear of your choice, skin on, and toss with 1/2 tablespoon lemon juice. Layer pear, parfait style, with a single-serve container of nonfat (0%) vanilla Greek yogurt, and 7 walnut halves, chopped. Sprinkle with cinnamon if desired. (Option: roast pear slices in the oven alongside rye flakes until soft.)

Peanut Butter Raspberry Toast

In a small bowl, sprinkle 1 cup fresh raspberries with a dash of cinnamon and mash slightly; set aside. Toast 1 slice (1 ounce) whole-grain rye bread. Spread with 1 tablespoon all-natural peanut butter and top with raspberries. Serve with 1 cup (8 ounces) skim milk. (Option: leave raspberries whole and enjoy separately.)

Cinnamon Raisin Oatmeal

In a small bowl, mix together 1/4 cup each unsweetened whey protein powder and rolled oats. Pour hot water over the mixture until you reach desired consistency (suggested amount: 1/4 cup water). Swirl in 2 teaspoons coconut oil, 2 tablespoons raisins, and a dash of cinnamon.

Open-Faced Egg Sandwich

Spread 1 slice (1 ounce) whole-grain rye bread with 1/4 of a ripe avocado. Top with 1/4 cup baby spinach leaves and 1 tomato, sliced. Top with 1 large egg (poached, scrambled, sunny-side up, or hard boiled, sliced). Enjoy with 1 small apple of your choice, skin on.

Strawberry Almond Smoothie

Chop 1 tablespoon unsalted raw or dry-roasted almonds; set aside. In a blender, combine a single-serve container of nonfat (0%) vanilla Greek yogurt, 1 cup frozen unsweetened strawberries, 1/4 cup unsweetened whey protein powder, and 1/4 cup water. Whip until smooth. Add almonds, 2 tablespoons rye flakes, 1/4 teaspoon cinnamon, and a handful of ice, and whip to desired consistency.

Apple Almond Cottage Cheese Toast

Chop 2 tablespoons almonds; set aside. Spread 1 slice (1 ounce) whole-grain bread with 1/2 cup low-fat cottage cheese and garnish with a dash of cinnamon. Top with 1 small chopped apple of your choice, skin on. Sprinkle with almonds.

Lunch Options

Open-Faced Tuna Sandwich

Chop 2 tablespoons unsalted raw or dry-roasted almonds. In a small bowl, mix 3 ounces chunk light tuna (canned in water, drained) with 1/2 teaspoon salt-free Italian herb seasoning, 1½ tablespoons balsamic vinegar, and chopped almonds. Spoon tuna mixture onto 1 slice (1 ounce) whole-grain rye bread. Serve with 1/2 cup each raw baby carrots and grape tomatoes. (Options: toast bread if desired, and use sliced or slivered almonds rather than whole, chopped.)

Mediterranean Tuna Salad

Rub or brush 1/2 cup eggplant chunks and 1/4 of medium red bell pepper, sliced, with 1 teaspoon extra-virgin olive oil. Place veggies on one end of a cookie sheet and place 2 rye crisps on the other end. Place cookie sheet in preheated 350°F oven for 5–10 minutes, checking every few minutes. Remove crisps when toasted and golden and veggies when soft. In a small bowl, whisk together 2 teaspoons extra-virgin olive oil, 2 teaspoons balsamic vinegar, and 1/4 teaspoon salt-free Italian herb seasoning. Add 4 ounces chunk light tuna (canned in water, drained) to bowl and toss with dressing. Place 1 cup mixed greens in a salad bowl. Top with eggplant, peppers, and tuna. Cut or crumble rye crisps over salad. (Option: leave rye crisps untoasted.)

Chicken and Veggie Pasta Salad

In a medium bowl, whisk together 2 teaspoons extra-virgin olive oil, 1 tablespoon balsamic vinegar, 1/4 teaspoon minced garlic, and 1 teaspoon lemon juice. Add 2 tablespoons minced onion, 1/4 cup each finely chopped kale, chopped mushrooms, and grape tomatoes, sliced in half, and 3–4 chopped fresh basil leaves. Fold in 3 ounces cooked boneless, skinless chicken breast, diced, and 1/2 cup cooked 100% whole-grain penne. Chill for at least 30 minutes (or overnight) and serve. (Option: to add another 20/20 Food, use whole-grain rye pasta.)

Lemony Lentil Salad

In a small bowl, toss 1/2 cup lentils (boiled, steamed vacuum sealed, or canned, drained and rinsed) with 1 teaspoon extra-virgin olive oil, 1/4 teaspoon minced garlic, and 1 tablespoon lemon juice; set aside. Toss 2 cups mixed greens with 2 teaspoons extra-virgin olive oil and 1 tablespoon balsamic vinegar. Transfer greens to a salad bowl, top with seasoned lentils, and garnish with 2 rye crisps, crushed.

Quick Black Bean Casserole

In a small saucepan over medium heat, sauté 1/4 teaspoon garlic in 1 tablespoon extra-virgin olive oil with 1/4 cup each chopped onion, mushrooms, carrots, and green bell peppers. Add 1/2 cup grape tomatoes, sliced in half, 1/2 cup spinach, 1/2 cup low-sodium vegetable broth, and a dash each cayenne pepper, black pepper, and crushed red pepper. Quickly bring to a boil, then reduce to a simmer and stir for 10–12 minutes. Stir in 1/3 cup cooked brown rice (fluffy, not packed) and 1/2 cup black beans and cook to heat through.

Open-Faced Tofu Pesto Sandwich

Spread 1 slice (1 ounce) whole-grain rye bread with 1 tablespoon basil pesto. Top with sliced or cubed extra-firm tofu (1/5 of a 14-ounce package) and cover with 1/4 cup greens of your choice and 5–6 rings of red onion. Serve with a side of 1/2 cup fresh grape tomatoes and 1 small tangerine.

Chickpea Lettuce Wraps

Preheat oven to 350°F. Toss 1/2 cup chickpeas (boiled or canned, rinsed and drained) with 2 teaspoons extra-virgin olive oil and 1/4 teaspoon minced garlic. Spread out on a cookie sheet and roast for 10 minutes. Fill 4 outer romaine leaves each with 1 tablespoon cooked, chilled whole-wheat couscous, roasted chickpeas, minced red onion, and chopped grape tomatoes.

Chicken Apple Walnut Salad

Chop 2 tablespoons walnuts; set aside. In a small bowl, whisk 2 teaspoons Dijon mustard with 1 teaspoon water, 1 teaspoon lemon juice, and 1/4 teaspoon minced garlic. Toss with 3 ounces cooked boneless, skinless chicken breast, diced. Place chicken salad over a bed of 1 cup fresh greens of your choice. Top with 1 small sliced apple of your choice, skin on. Sprinkle with walnuts and 1 crumbled rye crisp.

Open-Faced Moroccan Chicken Salad

In a small bowl, whisk together 2 teaspoons coconut oil, 1/4 teaspoon minced garlic, and 1/8 teaspoon ground cinnamon. Toss 3 ounces cooked boneless, skinless chicken breast, diced and chilled, and 2 tablespoons raisins in oil. Spoon chicken salad onto 1 slice (1 ounce) whole-grain bread (fresh or toasted).

Chickpea and Veggie Pasta Salad

In a medium bowl, whisk together 2 teaspoons extra-virgin olive oil, 1 tablespoon balsamic vinegar, 1/4 teaspoon minced garlic, and 1 teaspoon lemon juice. Add 2 tablespoons minced red onion, 1/2 cup baby spinach, 1/4 cup grape tomatoes, sliced in half, and 3–4 fresh basil leaves, chopped. Fold in 1/2 cup chickpeas (boiled or canned, rinsed and drained) and 1/2 cup cooked 100% whole-grain penne. Chill for at least 30 minutes (or overnight) and serve. (Option: to add another 20/20 Food, use whole-grain rye pasta.)

Shrimp and Veggie Lettuce Wraps

In a medium pan, stir together 1 tablespoon coconut oil, 1/2 teaspoon minced garlic, 1/4 cup low-sodium vegetable broth, and 1/8 teaspoon crushed red pepper. Add 1/2 cup each sliced mushrooms and chopped red bell pepper and sauté until mushrooms are slightly tender. Add 3 ounces cooked medium shrimp (peeled, deveined; frozen, thawed is OK) and heat through. Fill 2 large outer romaine leaves with veggie and shrimp mixture along with 1/2 cup cooked brown rice (fluffy, not packed).

Tofu and Spinach Tacos

In a medium pan, sauté 1 cup fresh baby spinach, 1/4 cup minced onion, and a dash each black pepper, cayenne pepper, and crushed red pepper in 1/4 cup low-sodium vegetable broth until onions are translucent. Add cubed extra-firm tofu (1/5 of a 14-ounce package) and heat through. Fill 2 taco-shaped whole-grain corn tortillas with veggie and tofu mixture and top with 1/4 of a ripe avocado, sliced.

LEMON PEPPER COD SALAD

In a small bowl, whisk 2 teaspoons Dijon mustard with 1 teaspoon water, 1 teaspoon lemon juice, and 1/4 teaspoon minced garlic. Toss with 3 ounces cooked, chilled, flaked cod filet. In a second small bowl, whisk together 2 teaspoons balsamic vinegar, 1 tablespoon extra-virgin olive oil, and 1/4 teaspoon ground black pepper. Add 1½ cups greens of your choice and toss to coat the leaves. Place greens in a salad bowl, top with cod salad, and serve with 2 rye crisps.

SHRIMP AND WILD RICE OVER SPINACH

In a medium pan, stir together 1 tablespoon coconut oil, 1/2 tea-spoon minced garlic, 1/4 cup low-sodium vegetable broth, and 1/8 teaspoon crushed red pepper. Add 1/2 cup each chopped red bell pepper and broccoli florets and sauté until broccoli is slightly tender. Add 3 ounces cooked medium shrimp (peeled, deveined; frozen, thawed is OK) and 1/2 cup cooked wild rice (fluffy, not packed) and heat through. Serve shrimp mixture over 1 cup baby spinach leaves. (Option: toss shrimp mixture with spinach, chill for at least 30 minutes, and serve cold.)

SPICY LENTIL CASSEROLE

In a small saucepan over medium heat, sauté 1/4 teaspoon garlic in 2 teaspoons extra-virgin olive oil with 1/3 cup each chopped onion, mushrooms, and broccoli florets. Add 1/2 cup grape toma-toes, sliced in half, 1/2 cup spinach, 1/2 cup low-sodium vegetable broth, and a dash each cayenne pepper, black pepper, and crushed red pepper. Quickly bring to a boil, then reduce to a simmer and stir for 8–10 minutes. Stir in 1/3 cup cooked brown rice and 1/2 cup lentils (boiled, steamed vacuum sealed, or canned, drained and rinsed) and heat through.

Chilled Lentil and Eggplant Salad

In a medium pan, sauté 1/2 teaspoon minced garlic, 1 cup cubed eggplant, 1/4 cup minced onion, and 1/4 teaspoon salt-free Italian herb seasoning in 1 tablespoon extra-virgin olive oil with 2 tablespoons low-sodium vegetable broth. Sauté until eggplant is tender. In a medium bowl, combine veggies with 1/3 cup cooked, chilled brown rice and 1/2 cup lentils (boiled, steamed vacuum sealed, or canned, drained and rinsed). Refrigerate at least 30 minutes or overnight.

Chicken and Wild Rice Lettuce Wraps

Toss 3 ounces cooked boneless, skinless chicken breast, diced and chilled, with 1 tablespoon extra-virgin olive oil and 1/2 teaspoon each minced garlic and salt-free Italian herb seasoning. Fill 2 large outer romaine leaves with chicken mixture and top each with 2 tablespoons cooked, chilled wild rice, minced red onion, and chopped grape tomatoes.

Tofu Spinach Walnut Pita

Chop 2 tablespoons walnuts; set aside. In a small bowl, whisk 2 teaspoons Dijon mustard with 1 teaspoon water, 1 teaspoon lemon juice, and 1/4 teaspoon minced garlic. Coat cubed extra-firm tofu (1/5 of a 14-ounce package) and 1 cup baby spinach leaves with mustard sauce. Stuff into half of a 100% whole-grain pita and garnish with walnuts.

Mediterranean Chicken Pita

In a small pan, sauté 1/2 teaspoon minced garlic in 2 teaspoons extra-virgin olive oil with 1/2 cup grape tomatoes, sliced in half, 1 cup baby spinach leaves, 1/4 cup minced onion, and 1/4 teaspoon salt-free Italian herb seasoning. Stuff into half of a 100% whole-grain pita with 3 ounces cooked boneless, skinless chicken breast, sliced.

Chicken and Veggie Tacos

In a small bowl, toss 1/4 cup each diced tomato and minced onion with 2 teaspoons lime juice and 1 tablespoon chopped cilantro; place in refrigerator to chill. In a medium pan, sauté 1 cup fresh baby spinach, 1/4 cup minced red bell pepper, and 1/4 cup sliced mushrooms in 2 teaspoons extra-virgin olive oil and 2 tablespoons low-sodium vegetable broth. Sauté until mushrooms are tender. Add 3 ounces cooked boneless, skinless chicken breast, diced, and heat through. Fill 2 taco-shaped whole-grain corn tortillas with veggie and chicken mixture and top with tomato mixture.

Dinner Options

Chicken with Garlicky Spinach and Corn

Bake or grill 3 ounces boneless, skinless chicken breast. Sauté 2 cups fresh spinach in 2 teaspoons extra-virgin olive oil with 1/4 teaspoon minced garlic. Steam or microwave 1/2 cup frozen corn and season with 1/8 teaspoon garlic powder (not garlic salt) and 1/4 teaspoon dried or 1/2 teaspoon fresh parsley. Serve cooked chicken with sides of spinach and corn.

Shrimp over Soba Noodles in Peanut Sauce

In a small pan, sauté 1/4 cup each broccoli florets, chopped red bell pepper, and onion with 1 cup baby spinach in 1/4 cup low-sodium vegetable broth. In a medium bowl, stir together 1 table-spoon all-natural peanut butter, 1/4 teaspoon fresh grated ginger, 1/4 teaspoon minced garlic, and a dash of crushed red pepper. Add 1/4 cup hot cooked soba noodles to bowl and toss until coated with peanut sauce. Place noodles on a plate and top with sautéed veggies and 3 ounces (start with 4 ounces raw) boiled or grilled medium shrimp (fresh, peeled, deveined or frozen, thawed).

Chicken with Almond Green Beans and Roasted Red Potatoes

Chop 2 tablespoons unsalted raw or dry-roasted almonds; set aside. Place 1/2 cup cubed Red Bliss potato, skin on, on a cookie sheet and bake in a preheated 350°F oven for 10 minutes or until tender. In a small bowl, whisk 2 teaspoons Dijon mustard with 1 teaspoon water, 1 teaspoon lemon juice, and 1/4 teaspoon minced garlic. Toss 1 cup steamed green beans in mustard sauce and garnish with almonds. Serve with 3 ounces cooked boneless, skinless chicken breast and roasted potatoes. (Option: use sliced or slivered almonds rather than whole, chopped.)

Shrimp and Veggie Stir-Fry

In a medium pan, stir together 2 teaspoons coconut oil, 1/2 teaspoon minced garlic, 1/4 cup low-sodium vegetable broth, and 1/8 teaspoon crushed red pepper. Add 3 ounces cooked medium shrimp (peeled, deveined; frozen, thawed is OK) and 1/4 cup minced onion and sauté 2 minutes. Add 1 cup greens of your choice and 1/2 cup broccoli florets and sauté until broccoli is slightly tender. Place sautéed veggies over a bed of 1/2 cup cooked brown rice (fluffy, not packed).

Chicken and Veggie Soup

In a medium saucepan, sauté 1/2 teaspoon minced garlic with 1/4 cup each minced onions and chopped carrots in 2 teaspoons extra-virgin olive oil until veggies are slightly tender. Add 1/2 cup low-sodium vegetable broth and 1/2 cup water, 1 teaspoon salt-free Italian herb seasoning, 1/2 cup grape tomatoes, sliced in half, and 1 cup spinach. Bring to a very brief boil, then reduce to a simmer for about 5–8 minutes. Add 1/2 cup frozen, thawed corn and 3 ounces cooked boneless, skinless chicken breast, minced. Stir for a few more minutes to heat through.

Ground Turkey in Ginger Peanut Sauce over Rice

In a small pan, sauté 1/4 cup each broccoli florets, chopped red bell pepper, and onion with 1 cup baby spinach in 1/4 cup low-sodium vegetable broth. In a medium bowl, stir together 1 tablespoon all-natural peanut butter, 1/4 teaspoon fresh grated ginger, 1/4 teaspoon minced garlic, and a dash of crushed red pepper. Add 3 ounces pan-browned extra-lean ground turkey and 1 tablespoon warm water and toss to coat with peanut sauce. Place 1/3 cup cooked brown rice (fluffy, not packed) on a plate and top with turkey, then veggies.

Baked Cod and Roasted Baby Brussels Sprouts

Chop 2 tablespoons walnuts; set aside. Place 4 ounces fresh cod in a shallow pan and 1 cup baby Brussels sprouts (fresh or frozen) on a cookie sheet. Place both in preheated 350°F oven and check often after 6 minutes. Remove cod when fish easily flakes with a fork and Brussels sprouts when golden and crisp on the outside and tender on the inside. Place Brussels sprouts on a bed of 1/4 cup cooked red quinoa and garnish with walnuts. Serve with cod and wedges of fresh lemon.

Lentils and Wild Rice over Spaghetti Squash

In a small bowl, whisk together 1 tablespoon extra-virgin olive oil, 1/4 teaspoon minced garlic, and a dash of cinnamon. Gently fold in 1/2 cup cooked lentils (boiled, steamed vacuum sealed, or canned, drained and rinsed); set aside. In a medium bowl, toss 1 cup cooked spaghetti squash with 1/2 cup baby spinach and 1/4 cup cooked wild rice. Place squash mixture on a plate and top with lentils.

Roasted Turkey with Warm Red Bliss Potato Salad

Chop 2 tablespoons unsalted raw or dry-roasted almonds; set aside. In a small bowl, whisk 2 teaspoons Dijon mustard with 1 teaspoon water, 1 teaspoon lemon juice, and 1/4 teaspoon minced garlic. Toss with 1/2 cup cubed Red Bliss potato, cooked (baked or boiled), skin on. Serve with 3 ounces oven-roasted boneless, skinless turkey breast and 1 cup steamed green beans, topped with almonds.

Lemony Chicken and Arugula Pasta

Over medium heat, sauté 1/4 teaspoon minced garlic in 2 teaspoons extra-virgin olive oil with 1/4 cup minced onion and 1/3 cup sliced mushrooms until onions are translucent. In a medium bowl, toss 3 ounces cooked boneless, skinless chicken breast, diced, with 1/2 cup 100% whole-grain penne, 1 cup fresh arugula, sautéed veggies, 1 teaspoon lemon juice, and 1/4 teaspoon fresh or 1/8 teaspoon dried lemon zest. (Option: to add another 20/20 Food, use whole-grain rye pasta.)

Spicy Turkey and Corn Stew

In a small saucepan over medium heat, sauté 1/4 teaspoon garlic in 1 tablespoon extra-virgin olive oil with 1/4 cup each chopped onion, mushrooms, carrots, and green bell pepper. Add 1/2 cup grape tomatoes, sliced in half, 1/2 cup spinach, 1/2 cup low-sodium vegetable broth, and a dash each cayenne pepper, black pepper, and crushed red pepper. Quickly bring to a boil, then reduce to a simmer and stir for 10–12 minutes. Stir in 1/3 cup frozen, thawed corn and 3 ounces pan-browned extra-lean ground turkey and heat through.

Mediterranean Seafood Pasta

In a medium pan, sauté 1/2 cup each cubed eggplant, chopped red bell peppers, chopped red onion, and sliced mushrooms in 2 teaspoons extra-virgin olive oil and 1/4 cup low-sodium vegetable broth with 1/2 teaspoon minced garlic and 1/4 teaspoon salt-free Italian herb seasoning, until veggies are slightly tender. Add 3 ounces baked cod, cut into chunks, and heat through. Serve over 1/2 cup cooked whole-grain pasta.

Roasted Vegetable Balsamic Chicken Salad

Place 1/4 cup each thinly sliced carrots, cubed eggplant, chopped red bell pepper, and frozen, thawed corn on a cookie sheet. Brush with 2 teaspoons extra-virgin olive oil and roast in a preheated 350°F oven for 10 minutes. Toss 2 cups mixed greens with 1 teaspoon extra-virgin olive oil, 2 teaspoons balsamic vinegar, and 1/4 teaspoon salt-free Italian herb seasoning. Transfer to a salad bowl, top with roasted vegetables and 3 ounces cooked boneless, skinless chicken breast, sliced.

Chicken and Veggie Stew

In a small saucepan over medium heat, sauté 1/4 teaspoon garlic in 2 teaspoons extra-virgin olive oil with 1/4 cup each chopped onion, zucchini, carrots, and green bell pepper. Add 1/2 cup grape tomatoes, sliced in half, 1/2 cup spinach, 1/2 cup low-sodium vegetable broth, and a dash each cayenne pepper, black pepper, and crushed red pepper. Quickly bring to a boil, then reduce to a simmer and stir for 10–12 minutes. Stir in 3 ounces cooked boneless, skinless chicken breast, diced, and 1/3 cup cooked brown rice (fluffy, not packed) and heat through.

Lentil and Brown Rice Soup

In a medium saucepan, sauté 1/4 cup each minced onions and chopped carrots and 1/2 cup cauliflower florets in 1 tablespoon extra-virgin olive oil with 1/2 teaspoon minced garlic until veggies are slightly tender. Add 1/2 cup low-sodium vegetable broth and 1/2 cup water, 1 teaspoon salt-free Italian herb seasoning, and 1/2 cup grape tomatoes, sliced in half. Bring to a very brief boil and then reduce to a simmer for about 10 minutes. Add 1/3 cup cooked brown rice (fluffy, not packed) and 1/2 cup lentils (boiled, steamed vacuum sealed, or canned, drained and rinsed). Stir for a few more minutes to heat through.

Almond Chicken Stir-Fry

Chop 2 tablespoons unsalted raw or dry-roasted almonds; set aside. In a medium pan, stir together 1/2 teaspoon minced garlic, 1/4 cup low-sodium vegetable broth, and 1/8 teaspoon crushed red pepper. Add 1/2 cup each greens of your choice, sliced mushrooms, and sliced carrots. Sauté until carrots are slightly tender. Add 3 ounces cooked boneless, skinless chicken breast, minced, and heat through. Place sautéed veggies and chicken over a bed of 1/3 cup cooked brown rice (fluffy, not packed). Garnish with almonds. (Option: use sliced or slivered almonds.)

Spinach and Cannellini Beans over Red Quinoa

In a medium pan, sauté 1½ cups baby spinach in 1 tablespoon extra-virgin olive oil with 1/4 teaspoon minced garlic, 1/4 teaspoon salt-free Italian herb seasoning, and 1/8 teaspoon crushed red pepper. Add 1/2 cup cannellini beans (boiled, steamed vacuum sealed, or canned, drained and rinsed) and heat through. Serve over 1/3 cup cooked quinoa (fluffy, not packed).

SALMON WITH SPINACH AND PISTACHIO RICE PILAF

Chop 1 tablespoon unsalted shelled pistachios; set aside. Place 4 ounces fresh salmon in a shallow pan in preheated 350°F oven and check often after 6 minutes. Remove salmon when fish easily flakes with a fork. In a medium pan, sauté 1 cup baby spinach and 2 tablespoons minced onion in 1/4 cup low-sodium vegetable broth with 1/2 teaspoon minced garlic. Add 1/3 cup cooked brown rice (fluffy, not packed) and pistachios and heat through. Serve with salmon and wedges of fresh lemon.

SPINACH AND SUNDRIED TOMATO CHICKEN

Sauté 1/4 cup minced onion, 1 cup baby spinach, 1/2 teaspoon minced garlic, and 4 finely chopped sundried tomatoes in 2 teaspoons extra-virgin olive oil and 2 tablespoons low-sodium vegetable broth until onions are translucent. Stir in 1/3 cup cooked brown rice (fluffy, not packed) and heat through. Serve mixture over 3 ounces cooked boneless, skinless chicken breast.

LENTIL AND BROWN RICE STUFFED PEPPER

Slice the top off 1 large red bell pepper and remove the inner seeds and membranes. Set pepper and top aside. Sauté 1/4 cup minced onion, 1 cup baby spinach, 1/2 teaspoon minced garlic, and 1/4 teaspoon salt-free Italian herb seasoning in 2 teaspoons extra-virgin olive oil until onions are translucent. Stir in 1/2 cup lentils (boiled, steamed vacuum sealed, or canned, drained and rinsed) and 1/3 cup cooked brown rice (fluffy, not packed) and remove from heat. Fill pepper with mixture, replace top, cover with foil, and bake in preheated 350°F oven for 15 minutes. Remove the foil and continue to bake for another 15 minutes (or until pepper is tender).

Snacks Options

Banana Walnut Muesli

In a small bowl, combine a single-serve container of nonfat (0%) vanilla Greek yogurt with 1/4 teaspoon ground cinnamon, 1/2 cup sliced banana, and 2 tablespoons each rolled oats and unsalted raw or dry-roasted walnuts, chopped. Chill in refrigerator at least 30 minutes. (Option: to add another 20/20 Food, use rye flakes in place of oats.)

Cherry Almond Parfait

Chop 2 tablespoons unsalted raw or dry-roasted almonds; set aside. Layer a single-serve container of nonfat (0%) vanilla Greek yogurt with 3/4 cup frozen, thawed unsweetened pitted cherries and 2 tablespoons rolled oats. (Option: to add another 20/20 Food, use rye flakes in place of oats.)

Basil Hummus with Apple Wedges

In a blender or food processor, purée 1/2 cup chickpeas, 2 teaspoons extra-virgin olive oil, 1/2 teaspoon minced garlic, 1 tablespoon lemon juice, and 3 fresh basil leaves. (Add water 1 tablespoon at a time, if needed, to thin hummus). Serve hummus with 2 rye crisps and 1 small chopped apple of your choice, skin on.

Kiwi Smoothie

In a blender, combine a single-serve container of nonfat (0%) vanilla Greek yogurt, 1 large chopped kiwi, 1/4 cup spinach, 1/4 cup unsweetened whey protein powder, and 2 tablespoons water. Whip until smooth. Add 1/4 of a ripe avocado, 1 tablespoon rolled oats, and a handful of ice, and whip to desired consistency.

Napa Valley Snack

Spread 2 rye crisps with 1 mini round cheese. Enjoy with a small pear of your choice, skin on, and 2 tablespoons unsalted raw or dry-roasted walnuts.

Peanut Butter Cinnamon Raisin Spread

Fold 1 tablespoon raisins and 1/4 teaspoon ground cinnamon into 1 tablespoon all-natural peanut butter. Spread onto 2 rye crisps and serve with a single-serve container of nonfat (0%) vanilla Greek yogurt.

Savory Cottage Cheese Crunch

Chop 2 tablespoons unsalted raw or dry-roasted walnuts; set aside. In a small bowl, combine 1/2 cup low-fat cottage cheese, 1/2 teaspoon minced garlic, 1 teaspoon Dijon mustard, and 1 cup chopped spinach. Toast 1 slice (1 ounce) 100% whole-grain bread. Spread with cottage cheese mixture and top with walnuts. Pair with 1/2 cup seedless grapes. (Option: enjoy walnuts separately.)

Blueberry Coconut Smoothie

In a blender, combine a single-serve container of nonfat (0%) vanilla Greek yogurt, 3/4 cup frozen unsweetened blueberries, 1/4 cup unsweetened whey protein powder, and 1/4 cup water. Whip until smooth. Add 2 teaspoons coconut oil, 1 tablespoon rye flakes, and a handful of ice, and whip to desired consistency.

Peanut Butter and Banana Crackers

Stir 1/4 teaspoon ground cinnamon into 1 tablespoon all-natural peanut butter. Spread onto 2 rye crisps and top with 1/2 cup sliced banana. Serve with 1 cup skim milk.

Pistachio Plum Cinnamon Yogurt

Chop 5 dried plums and stir into a single-serve container of nonfat (0%) vanilla Greek yogurt along with 2 tablespoons rye flakes, 1 tablespoon unsalted shelled pistachios, and 1/4 teaspoon ground cinnamon. (Option: chop or crush pistachios.)

Grape Muesli

In a small bowl, combine a single-serve container of nonfat (0%) vanilla Greek yogurt with 1/4 teaspoon fresh grated ginger, 1 cup seedless grapes (red, green, black, or a combo), sliced in half, and 1 tablespoon each rye flakes and unsalted sunflower seeds. Chill in refrigerator at least 30 minutes. (Option: replace ginger with a dash of cinnamon.)

Roasted Veggies and Hummus

Place 1/2 cup each sliced carrots and broccoli florets on a cookie sheet. Roast in preheated 350°F oven for 8–10 minutes or until tender. In a blender or food processor, purée 1/2 cup chickpeas, 2 teaspoons extra-virgin olive oil, 1/4 teaspoon minced garlic, and 1 tablespoon lemon juice. Serve hummus and roasted veggies with 2 whole-grain rye crisps. (Option: serve veggies raw, or roast, then chill veggies and serve cold.)

Pineapple Coconut Smoothie

In a blender, combine a single-serve container of nonfat (0%) vanilla Greek yogurt, 3/4 cup frozen unsweetened pineapple chunks, 1/4 cup unsweetened whey protein powder, and 1/4 cup water. Whip until smooth. Add 2 teaspoons coconut oil, 1 tablespoon rye flakes, and a handful of ice, and whip to desired consistency.

Mediterranean Munchies

Enjoy a snack of 1 large hard-boiled egg, 1 cup seedless grapes (red, green, black, or a combo), 2 whole-grain rye crisps, and 10 Mediterranean or Greek olives (green and black or just Kalamata). (Option: slice egg and place on top of rye crisps.)

Apple Gouda Toast

Chop 2 tablespoons unsalted shelled pistachios; set aside. Toast 1 slice (1 ounce) whole-grain rye bread and spread with 1 mini Gouda cheese. Top with pistachios and 1 small apple of your choice, skin on, sliced. (Option: enjoy pistachios separately.)

Strawberry Pistachio Parfait

Chop 2 tablespoons unsalted shelled or dry-roasted pistachios; set aside. Layer a single-serve container of nonfat (0%) vanilla Greek yogurt with 1 cup fresh or 3/4 cup frozen, thawed unsweetened strawberries, 2 tablespoons rolled oats, and the pistachios. (Option: to add another 20/20 Food, use rye flakes in place of oats.)

Sunny Peach Parfait

Layer a single-serve container of nonfat (0%) vanilla Greek yogurt with 1 medium fresh peach, sliced, or 3/4 cup frozen, thawed unsweetened sliced peaches, and 2 tablespoons each rye flakes and unsalted raw or dry-roasted sunflower seeds. (Option: replace rye flakes with rolled oats and pair parfait with green tea.)

Sunshine Snack

Enjoy a snack of 1 large hard-boiled egg, 1 medium orange, 2 whole-grain rye crisps, and 2 tablespoons unsalted raw or dry-roasted sunflower seeds. (Option: slice egg and place on top of rye crisps.)

Almond Plum Cheese and Crackers

Chop 2 tablespoons almonds and 3 dried plums. Melt 1 mini round cheese in the microwave. In a small bowl, fold almonds and plums into the cheese. Spread mixture onto 2 rye crisps.

Cinnamon Plum Cottage Cheese Crunch

Chop 2 tablespoons unsalted shelled pistachios; set aside. In a small bowl, combine 1/2 cup low-fat cottage cheese, 1/4 teaspoon ground cinnamon, and 5 chopped dried plums. Toast 1 slice (1 ounce) 100% whole-grain bread. Spread with cottage cheese mixture and top with pistachios. (Option: enjoy pistachios separately.)

APPENDIX C

The Management Phase: Foods and Portions

Prime Produce: Vegetables

Aim for: 1 cup fresh
      3/4 cup frozen
      1/2 cup all-natural tomato sauce

Artichokes

Asparagus

Beets

Bell peppers, all
   varieties

Broccoli

Brussels sprouts

Cabbage

Carrots

Cauliflower

Celery

Cucumbers

Eggplant

Fennel

Green beans

Greens, all varieties
   (arugula, baby
   mixed greens, bok
   choy, endive, field
   greens, radicchio,
   red leaf lettuce,
   romaine, baby
   spinach, watercress)

Kale

Mushrooms

Okra

Onion, all varieties

Radishes

Snow peas

Spaghetti squash

Sugar snap peas

Tomatoes, all varieties

Zucchini

Prime Produce: Fruit

Aim for: 1 small whole
      1 cup fresh (exception: bananas 1/2 cup sliced)
      3/4 cup frozen
      1/4 cup dried

Apples
Apricots
Bananas
Berries, all varieties
Cantaloupe
Cherries
Dried plums
Figs, fresh or dried
Grapefruit
Grapes, seedless, your choice (red, green, black)
Honeydew melon
Kiwi
Lemons
Limes
Mango
Nectarines
Oranges
Papaya
Peaches
Pears, all varieties
Pineapple
Plums
Raisins
Raspberries
Strawberries
Tangerines
Watermelon

Power Proteins:

Aim for: 4 ounces raw fish and poultry
      1/2 cup beans and lentils
      1/2 cup cottage cheese
      1 ounce natural cheese
      1 large egg or 1/2 cup egg whites
      1/5 of a 14-ounce container tofu
      1 cup skim milk
      1/4 cup whey protein
      6 ounces yogurt

Beans[†], all varieties (black, cannellini, pinto, red, etc.)
Catfish
Chickpeas, bagged or canned
Cheese, all natural (not processed or artificial)
Cod
Cottage cheese, low fat or nonfat
Chicken breast, boneless, skinless
Eggs, large, whole
Feta cheese
Flounder

continues ▶

[†]*Note: Canned beans are OK, but choose "no added salt" or "low-sodium" varieties and rinse them well.*

Power Proteins (*continued*):

Grouper

Haddock

Halibut

Lentils, bagged, steamed vacuum sealed, or canned

Liquid egg whites

Mahimahi

Mini round cheeses (roughly 70 calories each)

Salmon

Sea bass

Shrimp

Skim milk

Sole

Tilapia

Tofu, extra firm

Tuna, chunk light, canned in water

Turkey, ground, extra lean

Turkey breast, oven roasted, boneless, skinless

Yogurt—nonfat (0%) vanilla Greek yogurts (made with real sugar, not artificial sweetener)

Whey protein powder, unsweetened

Super Starches:

Aim for: 1/3–1/2 cup cooked whole grains
   (barley, corn, rice, pasta, etc.) and potatoes
   1 slice bread
   1/2 pita
   2 corn tortillas
   2 rye crisps

Barley

Breads, whole grain (includes whole-grain rye, whole wheat, or breads made with multiple whole grains)

Buckwheat

Bulgur

Cereal, whole grain, unsweetened (such as spoon-sized shredded wheat)

Corn

Corn tortillas, whole grain

Couscous, whole wheat

Oats, rolled

Pasta, whole grain

Pita, whole grain

Potatoes, all varieties, skin on

Quinoa, all varieties (golden, red, black)

Rice, whole grain (brown, wild)

Rye crisps, whole grain

Rye flakes, whole grain

Soba noodles, whole grain

Sweet potatoes

Fit Fat:

Aim for: 2 teaspoons oil or pesto
1/4 fresh avocado
2 tablespoons nuts or seeds
1 tablespoon nut butter
10 whole olives

Almonds
Avocado
Brazil nuts
Cashews
Coconut oil
Hazelnuts
Macadamia nuts
Olive oil, extra virgin

Nut or seed butters (peanut, almond, sunflower, etc.)
Olives, Mediterranean or Greek, your choice (green, black, Kalamata)
Peanuts

Peanut butter, all natural
Pesto, jarred
Pistachios, unsalted, shelled
Pumpkin seeds
Sunflower seeds
Walnuts

Other Phase 4 Necessities

Basil
Cilantro
Cinnamon
Cloves
Dijon mustard
Dill
Garlic
Ginger

Italian herb seasoning, salt free, dried
Nutmeg
Parsley
Pepper (black, cayenne, crushed red)

Vegetable broth, low sodium
Vinegar (balsamic, cider, red wine, white balsamic)
Zest (lemon, orange, lime)

BIBLIOGRAPHY

PART 1: Fundamentals of the 20/20 Diet

Introduction

Anderson, J., L. Young, and J. Roach. "Weight Loss Products and Programs." Colorado State University Extension, December 2008, accessed May 08, 2013. http://www.ext.colostate.edu /pubs/foodnut/09363.html.

"Gut Check: A Reference Guide for Media on Spotting False Weight Loss Claims." Bureau of Consumer Protection Business Center, January 2014, accessed June 25, 2014. http://www.business .ftc.gov/documents/0492-gut-check-reference-guide-media-spotting-false-weight-loss-claims.

Lee, Jeanne. "Diet Plan Review: Best Ways to Lose Weight." CBSNews, January 4, 2010, accessed May 08, 2013. http://www.cbsnews.com/8301-505145_162-51377880/diet-plan-review-best-ways -to-lose-weight/

Sumithran, P., L. A. Prendergast, E. Delbridge, et al. "Long-Term Persistence of Hormonal Adaptations to Weight Loss." *Obesity Research & Clinical Practice* 5 (October 2011): 15. doi:10.1016 /j.orcp.2011.08.082.

"The U.S. Weight Loss & Diet Control Market (12th ed.)." MarketData Enterprises, Inc. March 25, 2013. no. FS22. http://www.marketdataenterprises.com/DietMarket.htm.

"Top Four Reasons Why Diets Fail." *ScienceDaily,* January 03, 2013, accessed May 03, 2013. http://www.sciencedaily.com/releases/2013/01/130103192352.htm.

Chapter 1   What Makes This Diet Different

Cunningham, Eleese. "How Can I Help My Client Who Is Experiencing a Weight-Loss Plateau?" *Journal of the American Dietetic Association* 111, no. 12 (December 2011): 1966. doi:10.1016 /j.jada.2011.10.020.

Flegal, Katherine M., Margaret D. Carroll, Brian K. Kit, and Cynthia L. Ogden. "Prevalence of Obesity and Trends in the Distribution of Body Mass Index Among US Adults, 1999–2010." *JAMA: Journal of the American Medical Association* 307, no. 5 (February 1, 2012): 491–7. doi:10.1001 /jama.2012.39.

Levine, J. A. "Non-Exercise Activity Thermogenesis (NEAT)." *Best Practice & Research: Clinical Endocrinology & Metabolism* 16, no. 4. (December 2002): 679–702.

"Metabolism and Weight Loss: How You Burn Calories." Mayo Clinic, October 6, 2011. http://www.mayoclinic.com/health/metabolism/WT00006.

Ogden, Cynthia L., Margaret D. Carroll, Brian K. Kit, and Katherine M. Flegal. "Prevalence of Obesity and Trends in Body Mass Index Among US Children and Adolescents, 1999–2010." *JAMA: Journal of the American Medical Association* 307, no. 5 (February 1, 2012): 483–90. doi:10.1001/jama.2012.40.

Westerterp, K. R. "Diet induced thermogenesis." *Nutrition & Metabolism* 1, no. 1 (August 18, 2004): 5. doi:10.1186./1743-7075-1-5.

Chapter 2   A Diet That Defies Your Logic

Nackers, L. M., et al. "The Association between Rate of Initial Weight Loss and Long-Term Success in Obesity Treatment: Does Slow and Steady Win the Race?" *International Journal of Behavioral Medicine* 17 (2010): 161–7.

National Institutes of Health: National Heart, Lung, and Blood Institute; North American Association for the Study of Obesity. *The Practical Guide: Identification, Evaluation & Evaluation and Treatment of Overweight and Obesity in Adults.* October 2000. http://www.nhlbi.nih.gov/guidelines /obesity/prctgd_c.pdf.

Ozier, A., O. Kendrick, J. Leeper, et al. "Overweight and Obesity Are Associated with Emotion- and Stress-Related Eating as Measured by the Eating and Appraisal Due to Emotions and Stress Questionnaire." *Journal of the American Dietetic Association* 108, no. 1 (January 2008): 49–56. doi:10.1016/j.jada.2007.10.011.

PART 2: Prepping for Success

Chapter 3   Getting Out of Your Own Way

American Medical Association. "AMA Adopts New Policies on Second Day of Voting at Annual Meeting." News release, June 18, 2013. http://www.ama-assn.org/ama/pub/news /2013/2013-06-18-new-ama-policies-annual-meeting.page.

"Assessing Your Weight and Health Risk." National Heart, Lung, and Blood Institute, accessed May 08, 2013. http://www.nhlbi.nih.gov/health/public/heart/obesity/lose_wt/risk.htm.

"Imagery." American Cancer Society. November 1, 2008. http://www.cancer.org/treatment /treatmentsandsideeffects/complementaryandalternativemedicine/mindbodyandspirit/imagery.

Klein, S., D. B. Allison, S. B. Heymsfield, et al. "Waist Circumference and Cardiometabolic Risk: A Consensus Statement from Shaping America's Health: Association for Weight Management and Obesity Prevention; NAASO, The Obesity Society; the American Society for Nutrition; and the American Diabetes Association." *American Journal of Clinical Nutrition* 85, no. 5 (May 2007): 1197–202. http://www.nutrition.org/media/news/fact-sheets-and-position-papers//Waist%20 Circumference%20paper%20AJCN.pdf.

"Obesity, Halting the Epidemic by Making Health Easier at a Glance 2011." National Center for Chronic Disease Prevention and Health Promotion. May 26, 2011. http://www.cdc.gov /chronicdisease/resources/publications/aag/obesity.htm.

Prospective Studies Collaboration, Whitlock, G., Lewington, S., et al. "Body-Mass Index and Cause-Specific Mortality in 900,000 Adults: Collaborative Analyses of 57 Prospective Studies." *Lancet* 373, no. 9669. (March 28, 2009): 1083–96. doi:10.1016/S01410-6736(09)60318-4.

Sanches, F. M., C. M. Avesani, M. A. Kamimura, et al. "Waist Circumference and Visceral Fat in CKD: A Cross-Sectional Study." *American Journal of Kidney Disease* 52, no. 1 (July 2008): 66–73. doi:10.1053/j.akjd.2008.02.004.

"What is a healthy weight?" Rush University Medical Center, accessed June 18, 2013. http://www.rush.edu/rumc/page-1108048103230.html.

Chapter 4   Set the Right Goal

"Adolescent and School Health." Centers for Disease Control and Prevention, February 19, 2013, accessed May 14, 2013. http://www.cdc.gov/healthyyouth/obesity/facts.htm.

Begley, Sharon. "As America's Waistline Expands, Costs Soar." Reuters, April 30, 2012, accessed June 28, 2013. http://www.reuters.com/article/2012/04/30/us-obesity-idUSBRE83T0C820120430.

"Body Mass Index." Centers for Disease Control and Prevention, February 19, 2013, accessed August 8, 2014. http://www.cdc.gov/healthyweight/assessing/bmi/Index.html.

Jebb, S., A. Ahern, A. Olson, et al. "Primary Care Referral to a Commercial Provider for Weight Loss Treatment versus Standard Care: A Randomised Controlled Trial." *Lancet* 378, no. 9801 (October 22, 2011): 1485–1492. doi:10.1016/S0140-6736(11)61344-5.

Johnston, Craig A., Stephanie Rost, Karen Miller-Kovach, Jennette P. Moreno, and John P. Foreyt. "Incremental Benefit of Adherence in a Community-Based Weight Loss Program." *Journal of Clinical Lipidology* 7, no. 3 (May 2013): 244. doi:10.1016/j.jacl.2013.03.027.

Kullgren, Jeffrey T., A. B. Troxel, G. Loewenstein, et al. "Individual- versus Group-Based Financial Incentives for Weight Loss: A Randomized, Controlled Trial." *Annals of Internal Medicine* 158, no. 7 (April 2, 2013): 505–14.

"Obesity In Children and Teens." American Academy of Child & Adolescent Psychiatry, March 2011, accessed June 27, 2013. http://www.aacap.org/cs/root/facts_for_families/obesity_in_children_and_teens.

"Presentation: The Childhood Obesity Epidemic—Threats and Opportunities." Centers for Disease Control and Prevention, June 18, 2010, accessed June 27, 2013. http://www.cdc.gov/about/grand-rounds/archives/2010/06-June.htm.

Turner-McGrievy, G. M., and D. F. Tate. "Weight Loss Social Support in 140 Characters or Less: Use of an Online Social Network in a Remotely Delivered Weight Loss Intervention." *Transitional Behavioral Medicine*, January 2013.

Volpp, Kevin G., MD, PhD, Leslie K. John, MS, Andrea B. Troxel, ScD, et al. "Financial Incentive-Based Approaches for Weight Loss." *JAMA: Journal of the American Medical Association* 300, no. 22 (December 10, 2008): 2631–37. http://jama.jamanetwork.com/article.aspx?articleid=183047.

Chapter 5   Extinguish Your Fake Hunger

DR. PHIL'S 20/20 HUNGER AND FULLNESS SCALE

Chozen Bays, Jan. "Mindful Eating." *Psychology Today*, February 2009.
http://www.psychologytoday.com/blog/mindful-eating/200902/mindful-eating.

Paturel, Amy. "Conscious Eating for Better Body Image." Cleveland Clinic Wellness Institute,
September 9, 2009. http://www.clevelandclinicwellness.com/mind/BodyImage/Pages/
ConsciousEatingforBetterBodyImage.aspx.

"Weight Loss: Gain Control of Emotional Eating." Mayo Clinic, December 1, 2012.
http://www.mayoclinic.com/health/weight-loss/MH00025.

"Your Hunger Is Talking Learn to Listen." Cleveland Clinic Wellness Institute, accessed May 09, 2013.
http://www.clevelandclinicwellness.com/programs/NewGFFY/Pages/L4T4.aspx.

TOP SEVEN TRICKS FOR DEALING WITH FAKE HUNGER

American Academy of Sleep Medicine. "Evening blue light exposure linked to increased hunger."
ScienceDaily. www.sciencedaily.com/releases/2014/06/140602115916.htm (accessed June 10, 2014).

Boschmann, M., J. Steiniger, U. Hille, et al. "Water-Induced Thermogenesis." *Journal of Clinical
Endocrinology and Metabolism* 88, no. 12 (December 2003): 6015–9.

Creagan, Edward T. "Stress and Weight Gain." Mayo Clinic, July 23, 2011.
http://www.mayoclinic.com/health/stress/AN01128.

Hatzigeorgiadis A., et al. "Self-Talk and Sports Performance: A Meta-Analysis." *Perspectives on
Psychological Science*, July 2011. http://pps.sagepub.com/content/6/4/348.abstract.

Hogenkamp, P. S., E. Nilsson, V. C. NIlsson, et al. "Acute Sleep Deprivation Increases Portion Size
and Affects Food Choice in Young Men." *Psychoneuroendocrinology* S0306–4530, no. 13 (February 18,
2013). doi:10.1016/j.psyneuen.2013.01.012.

Li, J., N. Zhang, L. Hu, et al. "Improvement in Chewing Activity Reduces Energy Intake In One
Meal and Modulates Plasma Gut Hormone Concentrations in Obese and Lean Young Chinese
Men." *American Journal of Clinical Nutrition* 94, no. 3 (September 2011): 709–16. doi:10.3945
/ajcn.111.015164.

Markwald, R. R., E. L. Melanson, M. R. Smith, et al. "Impact of Insufficient Sleep on Total Daily
Energy Expenditure, Food Intake, and Weight Gain." *Proceedings of the National Academy of Sciences
of the United States of America* 110, no. 14 (April 2013): 5695–700. doi:10.1073/pnas.1216951110.

"Meditation: A Simple, Fast Way to Reduce Stress." Mayo Clinic, April 21, 2011.
http://www.mayoclinic.com/health/meditation/HQ01070.

"Obesity and Sleep." National Sleep Foundation, accessed May 16, 2013.
http://www.sleepfoundation.org/article/sleep-topics/obesity-and-sleep.

Papathanasopoulos, A., A. Rotondo, P. Janssen, et al. "Effect of Acute Peppermint Oil Administration
on Gastric Sensorimotor Function and Nutrient Tolerance in Health." *Neurogastroenterology and
Motility* 25, no. 4 (March 12, 2013): 263–71. doi:10.1111/nmo.12102.

Schieberle, P., V. Somoza, M. Rubach, L. Scholl, and M. Balzer. "Identifying Substances That Regulate
Satiety in Oils and Fats and Improving Low-Fat Foodstuffs by Adding Lipid Compounds with a

High Satiety Effect; Key Findings of the DFG/Aif Cluster Project 'Perception of Fat Content and Regulating Satiety: An Approach to Developing Low-Fat Foodstuffs.'" Technische Universitat Munchen, 2009–12. http://www.tum.de/en/about-tum/news/press-releases/short/article /30517/.

Spiegel, K., E. Tasali, P. Penev, and E. Van Cauter. "Brief Communication: Sleep Curtailment in Healthy Young Men Is Associated with Decreased Leptin Levels, Elevated Ghrelin Levels, and Increased Hunger and Appetite." *Annals of Internal Medicine* 141, no. 11 (December 7, 2004): 846–50.

St-Onge, M. P., A. L. Roberts, J. Chen, et al. "Short Sleep Duration Increases Energy Intakes but Does Not Change Energy Expenditure in Normal-Weight Individuals." *American Journal of Clinical Nutrition* 94, no. 2 (August 2011): 410–6. doi:10.3945/ajcn.111.013904.

"The Sleep Environment." National Sleep Foundation, accessed June 18, 2013. http://www.sleepfoundation.org/article/how-sleep-works/the-sleep-environment.

University of Rhode Island, Communications and Marketing. "URI Researcher Provides Further Evidence That Slow Eating Reduces Food Intake." News release, October 27, 2011. http://www.uri.edu/news/releases/?id=6019.

Yu, W. "Calm the Mind Before Bed." Cleveland Clinic Wellness Institute, September 8, 2009. http://www.clevelandclinicwellness.com/mind/BetterSleep/Pages/CalmtheMindBeforeBed.aspx.

Foods That Make You Hungry
Soda

Fowler, Sharon P., Ken Williams, Roy G. Resendez, et al. "Fueling the Obesity Epidemic? Artificially Sweetened Beverage Use and Long-Term Weight Gain." *Obesity* 16, no. 8 (June 05, 2008): 1894–900. doi:10.1038/oby.2008.284.

Piernas, C., D. F. Tate, X. Wang, and B. M. Popkin. "Does Diet Beverage Intake Affect Dietary Consumption Patterns? Results from the Choose Healthy Options Consciously Everyday (CHOICE) Randomized Clinical Trial." *American Journal of Clinical Nutrition* 97, no. 3 (January 30, 2013): 604–11. doi:10.3945/ajcn.112.048405.

Artificial Sweeteners

Feijo, F. M., C. R. Ballard, K. C. Foletto, et al. "Saccharin and Aspartame, Compared with Sucrose, Induce Greater Weight Gain in Adult Wistar Rats, at Similar Total Caloric Intake Levels." *Appetite* 60, no. 1 (January 2013): 203–7. doi:10.1016/j.appet.2012.10.009.

Raben, A., and B. Richelsen. "Artificial Sweeteners: A Place in the Field of Functional Foods? Focus on Obesity and Related Metabolic Disorders." *Current Opinion in Clinical Nutrition & Metabolic Care* 15, no. 6 (November 2012): 597–604. doi:10.1097/MCO.0b013e328359678a.

Swithers, S. E. "Artificial Sweeteners Produce the Counterintuitive Effect of Inducing Metabolic Derangements." *Trends in Endocrinology and Metabolism* 1043, no. 13 (July 3, 2013): 87–8. doi:10.1016/j.tem.2013.05.005.

White Starches and Sugars

Aller, E., I. Abete, A. Astrup, J. A. Martinez, and M. A. Baak. "Starches, Sugars, and Obesity." *Nutrients* 3, no. 3 (March 14, 2011): 341–69. doi:10.3390/nu3030341.

Processed Meats

Ifland, J. R., H. G. Preuss, M. T. Marcus, et al. "Refined Food Addiction: A Classic Substance Use Disorder." *Medical Hypotheses* 72, no. 5 (May 2009): 518–26. doi:10.1016/j.mehy.2008.11.035.

Fast Food

Jeffery, Robert W., Judy Baxter, Maureen McGuire, et al. "Are Fast Food Restaurants an Environmental Risk Factor for Obesity?" *International Journal of Behavioral Nutrition and Physical Activity* 3 (January 25, 2006): 2. doi:10.1186/1479-5868-3-2.

French Fries and Fried Chips

Anton, S. D., J. Gallagher, V. J. Carey, et al. "Diet Type and Changes in Food Cravings Following Weight Loss: Findings from the Pounds Lost Trial." *Eating and Weight Disorders* 17, no. 2 (June 2012): E101–108. http://www.ncbi.nlm.nih.gov/pubmed/23010779.

Crystal, S. R., and K. L. Teff. "Tasting Fat: Cephalic Phase Hormonal Responses and Food Intake in Restrained and Unrestrained Eaters." *Physiological Behavior* 89, no. 2 (July 17, 2006): 213–20. http://www.ncbi.nlm.nih.gov/pubmed/16846622.

Are You Being Manipulated? (Fast Food Advertising)

"Fast Food FACTS in Brief." Fast Food F.A.C.T.S., accessed May 03, 2013. http://www.fastfoodmarketing.org/fast_food_facts_in_brief.aspx.

Schlosser, Erin. "Americans Are Obsessed with Fast Food: The Dark Side of the All-American Meal." CBSNews, February 11, 2009, accessed May 03, 2013. http://www.cbsnews.com /2100–204_162-326858.html.

Chapter 6   Stock Up on Your 20/20 Foods

Foods with Potential Thermogenic Properties
Coconut Oil

Kasai, M., H. Maki, N. Nosaka, et al. "Comparison of Diet-Induced Thermogenesis of Foods Containing Medium- versus Long-Chain Triacylglycerols." *Journal of Nutritional Science and Vitaminology* (Tokyo) 48, no. 6 (2002): 536–40.

Marina, A. M., Y. B. Man, and Amin I. "Antioxidant Capacity and Phenolic Acids of Virgin Coconut Oil." National Center for Biotechnology Information, December 27, 2008. doi:10.1080 /09637480802549127.

Seaton, T. B., S. L. Welle, M. K. Warenko, and R. G. Campbell. "Thermic Effect of Medium-Chain and Long-Chain Triglycerides in Man." *American Journal of Clinical Nutrition* 44, no. 5 (November 1986): 630–4.

St-Onge, M. P., and P. J. Jones. "Physiological Effects of Medium-Chain Triglycerides: Potential Agents in the Prevention of Obesity." *Journal of Nutrition* 132, no. 3 (March 1, 2002): 329–32. http://jn.nutrition.org/content/132/3/329.full.

Green Tea

Diepvens, K., K. R. Westerterp, and M. S. Westerterp-Plantenga. "Obesity and Thermogenesis Related to the Consumption of Caffeine, Ephedrine, Capsaicin, and Green Tea." *AJP: Regulatory, Integrative and Comparative Physiology* 292, no. 1 (2006): R77-85. doi:10.1152/ajpregu.00832.2005.

Dulloo, A. G. "The Search for Compounds That Stimulate Thermogenesis in Obesity Management: From Pharmaceuticals to Functional Food Ingredients." *Obesity Reviews* 12. (2011): 866–83. doi:10.1111/j.1467-789X..2011.00909.x.

Dulloo, A. G., C. Duret, D. Rohrer, et al. "Efficacy of a Green Tea Extract Rich in Catechin Polyphenols and Caffeine in Increasing 24-h Energy Expenditure and Fat Oxidation in Humans." *American Journal of Clinical Nutrition* 70, no. 6 (December 1999): 1040–5.

Kokubo, Y., H. Iso, I. Saito, et al. "The Impact of Green Tea and Coffee Consumption on the Reduced Risk of Stroke Incidence in Japanese Population." *Stroke*, March 14, 2013. doi:10.1161.

Maki, K. C., M. S. Reeves, M. Farmer, et al. "Green Tea Catechin Consumption Enhances Exercise-induced Abdominal Fat Loss in Overweight and Obese Adults." *Journal of Nutrition* 139, no. 2 (February 2009): 264–70.

Nagao, T., Y. Komine, S. Soga, et al. "Ingestion of a Tea Rich in Catechins Leads to a Reduction in Body Fat and Malondialdehyde-Modified LDL in Men." *American Journal of Clinical Nutrition* 81, no. 1 (January 2005): 122–9.

Phung, O. J., W. L. Baker, L. J. Matthews, et al. "Effect of Green Tea Catechins with or without Caffeine on Anthropometric Measures: A Systemic Review and Meta-Analysis." *American Journal of Clinical Nutrition* 91, no. 1 (January 2010): 73–81. doi:10.3945./ajcn.2009.28157.

Rowe, C. A., M. P. Nantz, J. F. Bukowski, and S. S. Percival. "Specific Formulation of Camellia Sinensis Prevents Cold and Flu Symptoms and Enhances Gamma, Delta T Cell Function: A Randomized, Double-Blind, Placebo-Controlled Study." *Journal of the American College of Nutrition* 26, no. 5 (October 2007): 445–52.

Sano J., S. Inami, K. Seimiya, et al. "Effects of Green Tea Intake on the Development of Coronary Artery Disease." *Circulation Journal: Official Journal of the Japanese Circulation Society* 68, no. 7 (July 2004): 665–70.

Mustard

Cramer, Jenna M., Margarita Teran-Garcia, and Elizabeth H. Jeffery. "Enhancing Sulforaphane Absorption and Excretion in Healthy Men through the Combines Consumption of Fresh Broccoli Sprouts and a Glucoraphanin-Rich Powder." *British Journal of Nutrition* 107, no. 09 (May 2012): 1333–338. doi:10.1017/S0007114511004429.

Gregersen, N. T., A. Belza, M. G. Jensen, et al. "Acute Effects of Mustard, Horseradish, Black Pepper and Ginger on Energy Expenditure, Appetite, Ad Libitum Energy Intake, and Energy Balance in Human Subjects." *British Journal of Nutrition* 109, no. 03 (February 2013): 556–63.

Walnuts

Bullo, M., P. Casas-Agustench, A. Gomez-Flores, et al. "Acute Effects of Three High-Fat Meals with Different Fat Saturations on Energy Expenditure, Substrate Oxidation, and Satiety." *Clinical Nutrition* 28, no. 1 (February 2009): 39–45.

"Omega-3 Supplements: An Introduction." National Center for Complementary and Alternative Medicine, July 2009. http://nccam.nih.gov/health/omega3/introduction.htm.

Sabate, J., K. Oda, and E. Ros. "Nut Consumption and Blood Lipid Levels." *Archives of Internal Medicine* 170, no. 9 (May 10, 2010).

"USDA National Nutrient Database for Standard Reference," US Department of Agriculture, Agricultural Research Service, Nutrient Data Laboratory Home Page, Release 21, 2008. http://www.ars.usda.gov/ba/bhnrc/ndl.

West, S. G., A. L. Krick, L. C. Klein, et al. "Effects of Diets High in Walnuts and Flax Oil on Hemodynamic Responses to Stress and Vascular Endothelial Function." *Journal of the American College of Nutrition* 29, no. 6 (December 2010): 595–603.

OLIVE OIL

Bullo, M., P. Casas-Agustench, A. Gomez-Flores, et al. "Acute Effects of Three High-Fat Meals with Different Fat Saturations on Energy Expenditure, Substrate Oxidation and Satiety." *Clinical Nutrition* 28, no. 1 (February 2009): 39–45.

Marin, C., R. Ramirez, J. Delgado-Lista, et al. "Mediterranean Diet Reduces Endothelial Damage and Improves the Regenerative Capacity of Endothelium." *American Journal Clinical Nutrition* 93, no. 2 (February 2011): 267–74.

Ruano, C., P. Henriquez, M. Bes-Rastrollo, et al. "Dietary Fat Intake and Quality of Life: The SUN Project." *Nutrition* 10 (November 2011): 121.

Samieri, C., C. Féart, C. Proust-Lima, et al. "Olive Oil Consumption, Plasma Oleic Acid, and Stroke Incidence: The Three-City Study." *Neurology* 77, no. 5 (August 2011): 418–25.

FOODS THAT STICK TO YOUR RIBS

ALMONDS

Ketteler, Judi. "The Building Blocks of Flexibility." Cleveland Clinic Wellness Institute, October 2, 2009. http://www.clevelandclinicwellness.com/body/Flexibility/Pages/BuildingBlocksofFlexibility.aspx.

Mori, A. M., R. V. Considine, and R. D. Mattes. "Acute and Second-Meal Effects of Almond Form in Impaired Glucose Tolerant Adults: A Randomized Crossover Trial." *Nutrition & Metabolism* 8, no. 1 (January 28, 2011): 6. doi:10.1186/1743-7075-8-6.

"Nutrient Data for 12061, Nuts, Almonds." Agricultural Research Service National Agricultural Library. http://ndb.nal.usda.gov/ndb/foods/show/3615?fg=.

"Nuts, Grains & Seeds." Cleveland Clinic Wellness Institute. http://www.clevelandclinicwellness.com/Pages/CCWProductDetails.aspx?category=NutsandSeeds.

APPLES

Cleveland Clinic Wellness Editors. "An Apple a Day Really Can Keep the Doctor Away. Snack on Apples to Reduce Cholesterol and Fight Inflammation." Cleveland Clinic Wellness Institute. http://www.clevelandclinicwellness.com/DailyDose/archive/2011/10/25/Daily-Wellness-Tip-10-25-11.aspx.

Flood-Obbagy, J. E., and B. J. Rolls. "The Effect of Fruit in Different Forms on Energy Intake and Satiety at a Meal." *Appetite* 52, no. 2. (April 2009): 416–22. doi:10.1016/j.appet.2008.12.001.

Jamieson-Petonic, Amy, MEd, RD, CSSD, LD. "What's in Season: 5 Fall Foods to Eat Right Now." Cleveland Clinic Wellness Institute. http://www.clevelandclinicwellness.com/DailyDose/archive/2012/ 11/04/Seasonal-Foods-5-Fall.aspx.

Warren, Rachel M., MS. "Seasonal Eating for Your Body." Cleveland Clinic Wellness Institute, June 15, 2010. http://www.clevelandclinicwellness.com/food/SeasonalEating/Pages/SeasonalEatingforYourBody.aspx.

CHICKPEAS

Ball, M. J., C. M. Murty, and J. K. Pittaway. "Chickpea Supplementation in an Australian Diet Affects Food Choice, Satiety, and Bowel Health." *Appetite* 54, no. 2. (April 2010): 282–8. doi:10.1016/j.appet.2009.11.012.

Jamieson-Petonic, Amy, MEd, RD, CSSD, LD. "My 5 Favorite Foods for a Healthier 2012." Cleveland Clinic Wellness Institute. http://www.clevelandclinicwellness.com/DailyDose/archive/2012/01/09/favorite-foods-for-a-healthier-year.aspx.

Warren, Rachel M., MS, RD. "10 Snacks to Have on Hand At All Times!" Cleveland Clinic Wellness Institute, July 12, 2012. http://www.clevelandclinicwellness.com/food/FuelYourBody/Pages/10-snacks-to-have-on-hand-at-all-times.aspx.

COD

Borzoei, S., M. Neovius, B. Barkeling, A. Teixeira-Pinto, and S. Rossner. "A Comparison of Effects of Fish and Beef Protein on Satiety in Normal Weight Men." *European Journal of Clinical Nutrition* 60, no. 7 (July 2006): 897–902.

Cleveland Clinic Wellness Editors. "Top 10 Superfoods." Cleveland Clinic Wellness Institute, April 12, 2012. http://www.clevelandclinicwellness.com/food/FuelYourBody/Pages/top-10-superfoods.aspx.

"Mercury Levels in Commercial Fish and Shellfish" (chart). US Food and Drug Administration. http://www.fda.gov/Food/FoodborneIllness Contaminants/Metals/ucm115644.htm.

Wilk, J. B., M. Y. Tsai, N. Q. Hanson, J. M. Gaziano, and L. Djoussé. "Plasma and Dietary Omega-3 Fatty Acids, Fish Intake, and Heart Failure Risk in the Physicians' Health Study." *American Journal of Clinical Nutrition* 96, no. 4 (September 5, 2012): 882–8. http://www.ncbi.nlm.nih.gov/pubmed/22952185.

DRIED PLUMS (PRUNES)

Farajian, P., M. Katsagani, A. Zampelas. "Short-Term Effects of a Snack including Dried Prunes on Energy Intake and Satiety in Normal-Weight Individuals." *Eating Behaviors* 11, no. 3. (2010): 201–3. doi:10.1016/j.eatbeh.2010.02.004.

"Fitting Fiber In." Cleveland Clinic. http://my.clevelandclinic.org/heart/prevention/nutrition/fittingfiberin.aspx.

Provost, Jill. "20 Budget-Friendly Superfoods." Cleveland Clinic Wellness Institute, December 27, 2012. http://www.clevelandclinicwellness.com/food/smartfoodchoices/Pages/20-Budget-Friendly-Superfoods.aspx.

EGGS

Fallaize, R., L. Wilson, J. Gray, L. M. Morgan, and B. A. Griffin. "Variation in the Effects of Three Different Breakfast Meals on Subjective Satiety and Subsequent Intake of Energy at Lunch and Evening Meal." *European Journal of Nutrition* 52, no. 4 (June 2013): 1353–9. doi:10.1007/s00394-012-0444-z.

Pombo-Rodrigues, S., W. Calame, and R. Re. "The Effects of Consuming Eggs for Lunch on Satiety and Subsequent Food Intake." *International Journal of Food Sciences and Nutrition* 62, no. 6 (September 2011): 593–9. doi:10.3109/09637486.2011.566212.

Ronni, Chernoff, PhD, RD, FADA. "Protein and Older Adults." *Journal of the American College of Nutrition* 23, no. 6 (December 2004): 6275–305. http://www.jacn.org/content/23/suppl_6/627S.full.

Vander Wal, J. S., J. M. Marth, P. Khosla, K. L. Jen, and N. V. Dhurandhar. "Short-Term Effect of Eggs on Satiety in Overweight and Obese Subjects." *Journal of the American College of Nutrition* 24, no. 6 (December 2005): 510–15.

Wilson, L., R. Fallaize, J. Gray, L. M. Morgan, and B. A. Griffin. "Eggs at Breakfast Increase Satiety and Reduce the Subsequent Intake of Energy at Lunch and an Evening Meal Relative to Cereal or Croissant-based Breakfasts." *Proceedings of the Nutrition Society* 70, no. OCE6 (January 2011). doi:10.1017/S0029665111004502.

GREENS (ANY KIND OF LEAFY GREENS)

Cleveland Clinic Wellness Editors. "Top 10 Superfoods." Cleveland Clinic Wellness Institute, April 12, 2012. http://www.clevelandclinicwellness.com/food/FuelYourBody/Pages/top-10-superfoods.aspx.

Provost, Jill. "20 Budget-Friendly Superfoods." Cleveland Clinic Wellness Institute, December 27, 2012. http://www.clevelandclinicwellness.com/food/smartfoodchoices/Pages/20-Budget-Friendly-Superfoods.aspx.

Rolls, B. J., L. S. Roe, and J. S. Meengs. "Salad and Satiety: Energy Density and Portion Size of a First-Course Salad Affect Energy Intake at Lunch." *Journal of the Academy of Nutrition and Dietetics* 104, no. 10 (October 2004): 1570–76.

LENTILS

"35 Power Foods." Cleveland Clinic. http://my.clevelandclinic.org/heart/prevention/nutrition/35powerfoods.aspx.

Anderson, G. H., B. L. Luhovyy, R. C. Mollard, et al. "The Acute Effects of a Pulse-Containing Meal on Glycaemic Responses and Measures of Satiety and Satiation within and at a Later Meal." *British Journal of Nutrition* 108, no. 3. (August 2012): 509–17. doi:10.1017/S0007114511005836.

"Nutrient Data for 16070, Lentils, Mature Seeds, Cooked, Boiled, without Salt" (chart). *Agricultural Research Service National Agricultural Library.* http://ndb.nal.usda.gov/ndb/s/=&man=&lfacet=&format=&count=&max=25&offset=&sort=&qlookup=lentils.

"Nutrition Strategies to Reduce Your Risk of Cardiovascular Disease." Cleveland Clinic. http://my.clevelandclinic.org/heart/prevention/nutrition/strategies.aspx.

PEANUT BUTTER

"Know Your Fats." American Heart Association, May 1, 2013. http://www.heart.org/HEARTORG/Conditions/Cholesterol/Prevention TreatmentofHighCholesterol/Know-Your-Fats_UCM_305628_Article.jsp.

Reis, C. E., D. N. Robeiro, N. M. Costa, et al. "Acute and Second-Meal Effects of Peanuts on Glycaemic Response and Appetite in Obese Women with High Type 2 Diabetes Risk: A Randomized Cross-Over Clinical Trial." *British Journal of Nutrition* 109, no. 11 (November 5, 2012): 2015–023. doi:10.1017/S0007114512004217.

"The Whole Truth and Nutting But the Truth." Cleveland Clinic. http://my.clevelandclinic.org/heart/prevention/nutrition/nuts.aspx.

Pistachios

Dreher, M. L. "Pistachio Nuts: Composition and Potential Health Benefits." *Nutrition Reviews* 70, no. 4. (April 2012): 234–40. doi:10.1111/j.1753-4887.2011.00467.x.

Honselman, C. S., J. E. Painter, K. J. Kennedy-Hagan, et al. "In-Shell Pistachio Nuts Reduce Caloric Intake Compared to Shelled Nuts." *Appetite* 57, no. 2 (May 27, 2011): 414–7. doi:10.1016 /j.appet.2011.02.022.

Li, Z., C. Nguyen, A. Zerlin, H. Karp, et al. "Pistachio Nuts Reduce Triglycerides and Body Weight by Comparison to Refined Carbohydrate Snack in Obese Subjects on a 12-Week Weight Loss Program." *Journal of the American College of Nutrition* 29, no. 3 (June 2010): 198–203. http://www.ncbi.nlm.nih.gov/pubmed/20833992.

"Nuts about Nuts? For a Guilt-free Treat, Eat Pistachios. They Have Just 160 Calories per One-Ounce Serving." Cleveland Clinic Wellness Institute. http://www.clevelandclinicwellness.com /DailyDose/archive/2011/05/20/Daily_Wellness_Tip_5_20_11.aspx.

Raisins

"Add Color to Your Meals!" Missouri Department of Health and Senior Services. http://health.mo.gov/living/wellness/nutrition/.

Bays, H., K. Schmitz, A. Christian, et. al. "Raisins and Glucose: A Randomized, Controlled Trial." Presented at the American Diabetes Association's 72nd Annual Scientific Session, June 2012.

Puglisi, M. J., G. Mutungi, P. J. Brun, et al. "Raisins and Walking Alter Appetite Hormones and Plasma Lipids by Modifications in Lipoprotein Metabolism and Up-Regulation of the Low-Density Lipoprotein Receptor." *Metabolism* 58, no. 1 (January 2009): 120–8. doi:10.1016 /j.metabol.2008.08.014.

Rye

Isaksson, H., A. Rakha, R. Andersson, et al. "Rye Kernel Breakfast Increases Satiety in the Afternoon: An Effect of Food Structure." *Nutrition Journal* 10 (April 2011): 31. doi:10.1186/1475-2891-10-31.

Isaksson, H., I. Tillander, R. Andersson, et al. "Whole Grain Rye Breakfast: Sustained Satiety during Three Weeks of Regular Consumption." *Physiology and Behavior Journal* 105, no. 3 (October 28, 2011): 877–84. doi:10.1016/j.physbeh.2011.10.023.

Muralikrishna, G., and M. V. Rao. "Cereal Non-Cellulosic Polysaccharides: Structure and Function Relationship—An Overview." *Critical Reviews in Food Sciences and Nutrition* 47, no. 6 (2007): 599–610.

Van Dam, R. M., F. B. Hu, L. Roseberg, S. Krishnan, and J. R. Palmer. "Dietary Calcium and Magnesium, Major Food Sources, and Risk of Type 2 Diabetes in US Black Women." *Diabetes Care* 29, no. 10 (October 2006): 2238–43.

Tofu

"Soy (Glycine Max)." Mayo Clinic, September 1, 2012. http://www.mayoclinic.com/health/soy /NS_patient-soy.

Taku, K., K. Umegaki, Y. Sato, et al. "Soy Isoflavones Lower Serum Total and LDL Cholesterol in Humans: A Meta-Analysis of 11 Randomized Controlled Trials." *American Journal of Clinical Nutrition* 85, no. 4 (April 2007): 1148–56.

Williamson, D. A., P. J. Geiselman, J. Lovejoy, F., et al. "Effects of Consuming Mycoprotein, Tofu, or Chicken upon Subsequent Eating Behaviour, Hunger, and Satiety." *Appetite* 46, no. 1 (January 2006): 41–8.

Whey Protein

Ellis, V. and S. Pal. "The Acute Effects of Four Protein Meals on Insulin, Glucose, Appetite, and Energy Intake in Lean Men." *British Journal of Nutrition* 104, no. 8 (October 2010): 1241–8. doi:10.1017/S0007114510001911.

Markus, C. R., B. Olivier, and E. H. de Haan. "Whey Protein Rich in Alpha-Lactalbumin Increases the Ratio of Plasma Tryptophan to the Sum of the Other Large Neutral Amino Acids and Improves Cognitive Performance in Stress-Vulnerable Subjects." *American Journal of Clinical Nutrition* 75, no. 6 (June 2002): 1051–6.

"Whey Protein." Mayo Clinic, September 1, 2012. http://www.mayoclinic.com/ health/whey-protein /NS_patient-wheyprotein.

Yogurt

Cleveland Clinic Wellness Editors. "For a Healthier Yogurt, Go Greek. It Has Twice the Protein and Half the Sugar of the Sweet Type." Cleveland Clinic Wellness Institute. http://www .clevelandclinicwellness.com/DailyDose/archive/2012/09/14/Daily-Wellness-Tip-9-14-12.aspx.

Dougkas, A., A. M. Minihane, D. I. Givens, et al. "Differential Effects of Dairy Snacks on Appetite, but Not Overall Energy Intake." *British Journal of Nutrition* 108, no. 12. (December 2012): 2274–85. doi:10.1017/S0007114512000323.

Zeratsky, Katherine, RD, LD. "Is It Important to Include Probiotics and Prebiotics in a Healthy Diet?" Mayo Clinic. http://www.mayoclinic.com/health/probiotics/AN00389.

PART 3: The Three Phases of the 20/20 Diet

Chapter 7   Phase 1: The 5-Day Boost

Ford, E. S., and W. H. Dietz. "Trends in Energy Intake among Adults in the United States: Findings from NHANES." *American Journal of Clinical Nutrition* 94, no. 4 (April 2013): 848–53. doi:10.3945 /ajcn.112.052662.

Oliwenstein, Lori. "Caltech Researchers Pinpoint the Mechanisms of Self-Control in the Brain." California Institute of Technology, April 30, 2009.
http://www.caltech.edu/content/caltech-researchers-pinpoint -mechanisms-self-control-brain.

Pugh, Rachel. "Covertly Reducing Breakfast Calories Cuts Daily Food Intake." *Medscape Medical News*, May 13, 2013. http://www.medscape.com/viewarticle/804015.

"Reduction in Portion Sizes Led to Day-Long Reductions in Energy Intake." *Endocrine Today*, May 14, 2013. http://www.endocrinetoday.com/pda.aspx?rid=106781.

Meal Frequency Research

Cameron, J. D., M. J. Cyr, and E. Doucet. "Increased Meal Frequency Does Not Promote Greater Weight Loss in Subjects Who Were Prescribed an 8-Week Equi-Energetic Energy-Restricted Diet." *British Journal of Nutrition* 103, no. 8 (April 2010): 1098–101. doi:10.1017/S0007114509992984.

Ekmekcioglu, C., and Y. Toutiou. "Chronobiological Aspects of Food Intake and Metabolism and Their Relevance on Energy Balance and Weight Regulation." *Obesity Reviews* 12, no. 1 (January 2011): 14–25. doi:10.1111/j.1467-789X.2010.00716.x.

Farshchi, H. R., M. A. Taylor, and I. A. Macdonald. "Decreased Thermic Effect of Food after an Irregular Compared with a Regular Meal Pattern in Healthy Lean Women." *International Journal of Obesity and Related Metabolic Disorders* 28, no. 5 (May 2004): 653–60.

La Bounty, P. M., B. I. Campbell, J. Wilson, et al. "International Society of Sports Nutrition Position Stand: Meal Frequency." *Journal of the International Society of Sports Nutrition* 8, no. 4 (March 16, 2011): 4. doi:10.1186/1550-2783-8-4.

Ohkawara, K., M. A. Cornier, W. M. Kohrt, and E. L. Melanson. "Effects of Increased Meal Frequency on Fat Oxidation and Perceived Hunger." *Obesity* (Silver Spring) 21, no. 2 (February 2013): 336–43. doi:10.1002/oby.20032.

Allergy Replacements

"About Food Allergies." Food Allergy Research & Education, accessed June 19, 2013. http://www.foodallergy.org/about-food-allergies.

Li, James. "What's the Difference between a Food Intolerance and Food Allergy?" Mayo Clinic, June 3, 2011. http://www.mayoclinic.com/health/food-allergy/AN01109.

Coffee Drinking Statistics

Neal, R. "Caffeine Nation." CBS News, February 11, 2009. http://www.cbsnews.com/8301-3445_162-529388.html.

Saad, L. "Nearly Half of Americans Drink Soda Daily." GALLUP, July 23, 2012. http://www.gallup.com/poll/156116/nearly-half-americans-drink-soda-daily.aspx.

Phase 1 Seasonings
Garlic

Elkayam, A., D. Mirelman, T. Miron, et al. "The Effects of Allicin on Weight in Fructose-Induced Hyperinsulinemic, Hyperlipidemic, Hypertensive Rats." *American Journal of Hypertension.* 16. no. 12. (2003): 1053–6.

"Herbs at a Glance: Garlic." National Center for Complementary and Alternative Medicine. NCCAM pub. no. D274 (April 2012). http://nccam.nih.gov/health/garlic/ataglance.htm.

Lee, M. S., I. H. Kim, C. T. Kim, and Y. Kim. "Reduction of Body Weight by Dietary Garlic Associated with an Increase in Uncoupling Protein mRNA Expression and Activation of AMP-Activated Protein Kinase in Diet-Induced Obese Mice." *Journal of Nutrition* 141, no. 11 (November 2011): 1947–53. doi:10.3945/jn.111.146050.

Parker-Pope, Tara. "Unlocking the Benefits of Garlic." *New York Times*, October 15, 2007, accessed April 29, 2013. http://well.blogs.nytimes.com/2007/10/15/unlocking-the-benefits-of-garlic.

Cinnamon

Almer L. O., O. Bjorgell, G. Darwiche, et al. "Effects of 1 and 3 g Cinnamon on Gastric Emptying, Satiety, and Postprandial Blood Glucose, Insulin, Glucose-Dependent Insulinotropic Polypeptide, Glucagon-like Peptide 1, and Ghrelin Concentrations in Healthy Subjects." *American Journal of Clinical Nutrition* 89, no. 3 (2009): 815–21. doi:10.3945/ajcn.2008.26807.

Anderson, R. A. "Chromium and Polyphenols from Cinnamon Improve Insulin Sensitivity." *Proceedings of the Nutrition Society* 67, no. 1 (February 2008): 48–53. doi:10.1017/S0029665108006010.

Bonci, Leslie, and Selene Yeager. *The Active Calorie Diet: Eat More, Burn More, Lose More with Our Breakthrough 4-Week Program*. Emmaus, PA: Rodale, 2011.

Gruenwald, J., J. Freder, and N. Armbruester. "Cinnamon and Health." *Critical Reviews in Food Science and Nutrition* 50, no. 9 (October 2010): 822–34. doi:10.1080/10408390902773052.

Magistrelli, A., and J. C. Chezem. "Effect of Ground Cinnamon on Postprandial Blood Glucose Concentration in Normal-Weight and Obese Adults." *Journal of the Academy of Nutrition and Dietetics* 112, no. 11. (November 2012): 1806–09. doi:10.1016/j.jand.2012.07.037.

LEMON

Higdon, Jane. "Vitamin C." Linus Pauling Institute, Oregon State University, January 2006, updated and reviewed November 2009, accessed April 29, 2013. http://lpi.oregonstate.edu/infocenter/vitamins/vitaminC/.

Johnston, C. S. "Strategies for Healthy Weight Loss: From Vitamin C to the Glycemic Response." *Journal of the American College of Nutrition* 24, no. 3. (2005): 158–65.

Johnston, C. S., C. Corte, and P. D. Swan. "Marginal Vitamin C Status Is Associated with Reduced Fat Oxidation during Submaximal Exercise in Young Adults." *Nutrition & Metabolism* 3. (August 31, 2006): 35.

Juraschek, S. P., E. Guallar, L. J. Appel, and E. R. Miller III. "Effects of Vitamin C Supplementation on Blood Pressure: A Meta-Analysis of Randomized Controlled Trials." *American Journal of Clinical Nutrition* 95, no 5. (May 2012): 1079–88. doi:10.3945/ajcn.111.027995.

Pan, Min-Hsiung, Ching-Shu Lai, and Chi-Tang Ho. "Anti-inflammatory Activity of Natural Dietary Flavonoids." *Food & Function* 1, no. 1 (October 2010): 15. doi:10.1039/c0fo00103a.

Chapter 8   Phase 2: The 5-Day Sustain

NEW PHASE 2 FOODS: BENEFITS

"Beta-carotene." Natural Medicines Comprehensive Database, July 2011. http://www.nlm.nih.gov/medlineplus/druginfo/natural/999.html.

"Carbohydrates." Harvard School of Public Health Nutrition Source. http://www.hsph.harvard.edu/nutritionsource/carbohydrates.

"Carbohydrates." National Institutes of Health, May 2012. http://www.nlm.nih.gov/medlineplus/ency/article/002469.htm.

Dietary Reference Intakes for Energy, Carbohydrate, Fiber, Fat, Fatty Acids, Cholesterol, Protein, and Amino Acids. Washington, DC: National Academies Press, 2005.

Godman, H. "Lycopene-Rich Tomatoes Linked to Lower Stroke Risk." *Harvard Health Blog*, October 10, 2012. http://www.health.harvard.edu/blog/lycopene-rich-tomatoes-linked-to -lower-stroke-risk-201210105400.

Hwang, E. S., and P. E. Bowen. "Can the Consumption of Tomatoes or Lycopene Reduce Cancer Risk?" *Integrative Cancer Therapies* 1, no. 2 (June 2002): 121–32.

"Improving Your Health with Fiber." Cleveland Clinic, April, 2010. http://my.clevelandclinic.org/ healthy_living/nutrition/hic_improving_your_health_with_fiber.aspx.

"Lycopene." Natural Medicines Comprehensive Database, August 2011. http://www.nlm.nih.gov/medlineplus/druginfo/natural/554.html.

Provost, Jill. "20 Budget-Friendly Superfoods." Cleveland Clinic Wellness Institute, December 27, 2012. http://www.clevelandclinicwellness.com/food/smartfoodchoices/Pages/20-Budget-Friendly-Superfoods.aspx.

Sensible Splurging

De Witt Huberts, J. C., C. Evers, and D. T. De Ridder. "Double Trouble: Restrained Eaters Do Not Eat Less and Feel Worse." *Psychology & Health* 28, no. 6 (June 2013): 686–700.

Jakubowicz, D., O. Froy, J. Wainstein, and M. Boaz. "Meal Timing and Composition Influence Ghrelin Levels, Appetite Scores, and Weight Loss Maintenance in Overweight and Obese Adults." *Steroids* 77, no. 4 (March 10, 2012): 323–31. doi:10.1016/j.steroids.2011.12.006.

Redden, J. P., and K. L. Haws. "Healthy Satiation: The Role of Decreasing Desire in Effective Self-Control." *Journal of Consumer Research* 39, no. 5 (February 2013): 1100–14.

Truong, G., D. J. Turk, and T. C. Handy. "An Unforgettable Apple: Memory and Attention for Forbidden Objects." *Cognitive, Affective & Behavioral Neuroscience* (epub), May 24, 2013.

Van Kleef, E., M. Shimizu, and B. Wansink. "Just a Bite: Considerably Smaller Snack Portions Satisfy Delayed Hunger and Craving." *Food Quality and Preference* 27, no. 1 (January 2013): 96–100. doi:10.1016/j.foodqual.2012.06.008.

Chapter 9 Phase 3: The 20-Day Attain

Coping with Emotional Triggers

Herbert, Cornelia, Paul Pauli, and Paul A. Breslin. "Oral Perceptions of Fat and Taste Stimuli Are Modulated by Affect and Mood Induction." *PLoS One* 8, no. 6 (2013).

Eating Out

California Pizza Kitchen

"Menu—Roasted Veggie Salad." California Pizza Kitchen. http://www.cpk.com/menu/#Salads.

Cheesecake Factory

"Seared Tuna Tataki Salad." Cheesecake Factory. http://www.thecheesecakefactory.com/menu/Salads/seared_tuna _tataki_salad.

"Veggie Burger." Cheesecake Factory. http://www.thecheesecakefactory.com/menu/glamburgers/veggie_burger.

Chili's

"Lighter Choices— Mango-Chile Chicken & Caribbean Salad" Chile's. http://www.chilis.com/EN/Pages/menuitem.aspx?CatId=C918423.

"Salads." Chile's. http://www.chilis.com/EN/Pages/menuitem.aspx?CatId=C918423.

Chipotle

"Menu—Salad." Chipotle Mexican Grill. http://www.chipotle.com/en-us/menu/menu.aspx.

El Pollo Loco

"Fire-Grilled Skinless Breast Meal—Nutrition Facts." El Pollo Loco. http://m.elpolloloco.com
/our-food/#/nutrition/8df1244a-6e74-4bc9-9258-17e028654fc6/Fire-Grilled Skinless Breast
Meal.

Macaroni Grill

"Nutrition Information—Grilled Chicken Spiedini." Romano's Macaroni Grill (last updated April
2013). http://www.macaronigrill.com/docs/nutritional/nutritional-menu.pdf.

Olive Garden

"Nutrition—Lighter Italian Fare." Olive Garden Italian Restaurant. http://www.olivegarden.com
/Menu/Nutrition/.

"Nutrition—Soups & Salads." Olive Garden Italian Restaurant. http://www.olivegarden.com/Menu
/Nutrition/.

Outback Steakhouse

"Nutrition Information, Total Meal—California Chicken Salad." Outback Steakhouse (last updated
January 2013). http://www.outback.com/menu/nutritionitem.aspx?id=4565.

Panera Bread

"Access into Panera's Hidden Menu." Panera Bread. http://mypanera.panerabread.com/articlestips
/article/access-into-paneras-hidden-menu.

PF Chang's

"Nutrition Information—Buddha's Feast." PF Chang's. http://www.pfchangs.com/menu
/nutritionalinfo.aspx.

Qdoba

"Menu—Taco Salad." Qdoba Mexican Grill. http://www.qdoba.com/menu-nutrition
/taco-salad-menu-nutrition.

Starbucks

"Protein Bistro Box." Starbucks Coffee. http://www.starbucks.com/menu/food/bistro-boxes
/protein?foodZone=9999.

PART 4: Your Body's Capacity for Change

Chapter 10   The 30-Second Burn Burst Exercise Program

Baar, K. "To Perform Your Best: Work Hard Not Long." *Journal of Physiology* 575, pt. 3 (September 15,
2006): 690.

Bangsbo J., Nielsen J. J., Mohr M., et al. "Performance Enhancements and Muscular Adaptations of a
16-Week Recreational Football Intervention for Untrained Women." *Scandinavian Journal of Medicine
& Science in Sports*, (2009): 24–30. http://www.ncbi.nlm.nih.gov/pubmed/19954496.

Dwyer, T., A. L. Ponsonby, O. C. Ukoumunne, et al. "Association of Change in Daily Step Count
Over Five Years with Insulin Sensitivity and Adiposity: Population Based Cohort Study." *BMJ:
British Medical Journal* 342 (January 13, 2011): c7249. doi:10.1136/bmj.c7249.

Gibala M. J., J. P. Little, M. van Essen, et al. "Short-Term Sprint Interval versus Traditional Endurance Training: Similar Initial Adaptations in Human Skeletal Muscle and Exercise Performance." *Journal of Physiology* 575 (September 15, 2006): 901–11.

"Global Recommendations on Physical Activity for Health." World Health Organization, 2011. http://www.who.int/dietphysicalactivity/physical-activity-recommendations-18-64years.pdf.

Hazell, T. J., R. E. Macpherson, B. M. Gravelle, and P. W. Lemon. "10 or 30-s Sprint Interval Training Bouts Enhance Both Aerobic and Anaerobic Performance." *European Journal of Applied Physiology* 110, no. 1 (September 2010): 153–60. doi:10.1007/s00421-010-1474-y.

Lemon, Marc, Dirk Moelants, Matthias Varewyck, et al. "Activating and Relaxing Music Entrains the Speed of Beat Synchronized Walking." *Public Library of Science One* 8, no. 7 (July 10, 2013). doi:10.1371/journal.pone.0067932.

Macfarlane, Duncan J., Lynne H. Taylor, and Thomas F. Cuddihy. "Very Short Intermittent vs Continuous Bouts of Activity in Sedentary Adults." *Preventive Medicine* 43, no. 4 (October 2006): 332–6. (Accessed June 11, 2014). doi:10.1016/j.ypmed.2006.06.002.

Pal, S., C. Cheng, and S. Ho. "The Effect of Two Different Health Messages on Physical Activity Levels and Health in Sedentary, Overweight, Middle-Aged Women." *BMC Public Health Journal* 11 (March 31, 2011): 204. doi:10.1186/1471-2458-11-204.

"Physical Activity Guidelines for Americans." US Department of Health and Human Services, October, 2008. http://www.health.gov/paguidelines/guidelines/summary.aspx.

Stokes K. A., M. E. Nevill, G. M. Hall, and H. K. Lakomy. "The Time Course of the Human Growth Hormone Response to a 6 s and a 30 s Cycle Ergometer Sprint." *Journal of Sports Science* 20, no. 6 (June 2002): 487–94.

Teta, Jade, and Keoni Teta. "Hormonal Weight Loss: Is There Such a Thing as the 'Metabolic Effect'?" 2005. http://www.sprinttraining.co.uk/Documents/Hormonal_Weight_Loss.pdf.

"The Surgeon General's Vision for a Healthy and Fit Nation." US Department of Health and Human Services, Office of the Surgeon General, January 2010. http://www.surgeongeneral.gov/initiatives/healthy-fit-nation/obesityvision2010.pdf.

Ziemann, E., T. Grzywacz, M. Luszcyk, et al. "Aerobic and Anaerobic Changes with High-Intensity Interval Training in Active College-Aged Men." *Journal of Strength and Conditioning Research* 25, no. 4 (April 2011): 1104–12. doi:10.1519/JSC.0b013e3181d09ec9.

RPE Scale

"Perceived Exertion (Borg Rating of Perceived Exertion Scale)." Centers for Disease Control and Prevention, March 30, 2011, accessed May 08, 2013. http://www.cdc.gov/physicalactivity/everyone/measuring/exertion.html.

"Rated Perceived Exertion (RPE) Scale." Cleveland Clinic, accessed May 08, 2013. http://my.clevelandclinic.org/heart/prevention/exercise/rpe.aspx.

HIIT and HIRT Exercise

Heydari, M., J. Freund, and S. H. Boutcher. "The Effect of High-Intensity Intermittent Exercise on Body Composition of Overweight Young Males." *Journal of Obesity* 2012 (April 2012).

Little, J. P., A. Safdar, G. P. Wilkin, M. A. Tarnopolsky, and M. J. Gibala. "A Practical Model of Low-Volume High-Intensity Interval Training Induces Mitochondrial Biogenesis in Human

Skeletal Muscle: Potential Mechanisms." *Journal of Physiology* 588, no. 6 (March 15, 2010): 1011–22. doi:10.1113/jphysiol.2009.181743.

Paoli, A., T. Moro, G. Marcolinet, et al. "High-Intensity Interval Resistance Training (HIRT) Influences Resting Energy Expenditure and Respiratory Ratio in Non-Dieting Individuals." *Journal of Translational Medicine* 10 (November 24, 2012): 237. doi:10.1186/1479-5876-10-237.

Roy, Brad. "High-Intensity Interval Training: Efficient, Effective, and a Fun Way to Exercise." *ACSM'S Health & Fitness Journal* 17, no. 3. (May/June 2013): 3. doi:10.1249/FIT.0b013e31828cb21c.

Shiraev, T., and G. Barclay. "Evidence Based Exercise—Clinical Benefits of High Intensity Interval Training." *Australian Family Physician* 41, no. 12 (December 2012): 960–2.

Tjonna, A. E., I. M. Leinan, A. T. Bartnes, et al. "Low- and High-Volume of Intensive Endurance Training Significantly Improves Maximal Oxygen Uptake after 10-Weeks of Training in Healthy Men." *PLoS ONE* 8, no. 5 (May 2013).

Trapp, E. G., D. J. Chisholm, J. Freund, and S. H. Boutcher. "The Effects of High-Intensity Intermittent Exercise Training on Fat Loss and Fasting Insulin Levels of Young Women." *International Journal of Obesity* 32, no. 4 (2008): 684–91. doi:10.1038/sj.ijo.0803781.

Tresierras, M. A., and G. J. Balady. "Resistance Training in the Treatment of Diabetes and Obesity: Mechanisms and Outcomes." *Journal of Cardiopulmonary Rehabilitation & Prevention* 29, no. 2 (March/April 2009): 67–75.

Verial, Damon. "Workout Routines for High Intensity Resistance Training." AZ Central Healthy Living, accessed May 09, 2013. http://healthyliving.azcentral.com/workout-routines-high-intensity-resistance-training-1863.html.

REDUCING MUSCLE SORENESS

Ahmaidi, Said, Pascale Granier, Zohra Taoutaou, et al. "Effects of Active Recovery on Plasma Lactate and Anaerobic Power following Repeated Intensive Exercise." *Medicine & Science in Sports & Exercise* 28, no. 4 (April 1996): 450–6. doi:10.1097/00005768-199604000-00009.

Micklewright, D. P., R. Beneke, V. Gladwell, and M. H. Sellens. "Blood Lactate Removal Using Combined Massage and Active Recovery." *Medicine & Science in Sports & Exercise* 35, supplement 1 (May 2003): S317. doi:10.1097/00005768-200305001-01755.

Chapter 11   When Your Body Won't Follow Your Mind: Are You Resistant to Weight Loss?

WEIGHT LOSS RESISTANCE

Block, J. P., Y. He, A. M. Zaslavsky, L. Ding, and J. Z. Ayanian. "Psychosocial Stress and Change in Weight Among US Adults." *American Journal of Epidemiology* 170, no. 2 (2009): 181–92. doi:10.1093/aje/kwp104.

Davila, David G. "Food and Sleep." National Sleep Foundation, December 2009, accessed May 09, 2013. http://www.sleepfoundation.org/article/sleep-topics/food-and-sleep.

Dokken, Betsy B., and Tsu-Shuen Tsao. "The Physiology of Body Weight Regulation: Are We Too Efficient for Our Own Good?" *Diabetes Spectrum* 20, no. 3 (July 2007): 166–70. doi:10.2337/diaspect.20.3.166.

Donga, E., M. Van Dijk, J. G. Van Dijk, et al. "A Single Night of Partial Sleep Deprivation Induces Insulin Resistance in Multiple Metabolic Pathways in Healthy Subjects." *Journal of Clinical Endocrinology & Metabolism* 95, no. 6 (June 2010): 2963–68. doi:10.1210/jc.2009-2430.

Leproult, R., G. Copinschi, O. Buxton, and E. Van Cauter. "Sleep Loss Results in an Elevation of Cortisol Levels the Next Evening." *Sleep* 20, no. 10 (October 1997): 865–70.

Lovallo, W. R. "Caffeine Stimulation of Cortisol Secretion Across the Waking Hours in Relation to Caffeine Intake Levels." *Psychosomatic Medicine* 67, no. 5 (2005): 734–39. doi:10.1097/01 .psy.0000181270.20036.06.

Rooyackers, Olav E., and K. Sreekumaran Nair. "Hormonal Regulation of Human Muscle Protein Metabolism." *Annual Review of Nutrition* 17, no. 1 (1997): 457–85. doi:10.1146/annurev .nutr.17.1.457.

Schmid, Sebastian M., Manfred Hallschmid, Kamila Jauch-Chara, Jan Born, and Bernd Schultes. "A Single Night of Sleep Deprivation Increases Ghrelin Levels and Feelings of Hunger in Normal-weight Healthy Men." *Journal of Sleep Research* 17, no. 3 (2008): 331–4. doi:10.1111 / j.1365-2869.2008.00662.x.

Tomiyama, A. J., T. Mann, D. Vinas, et al. "Low Calorie Dieting Increases Cortisol." *Psychosomatic Medicine* 72, no. 4 (2010): 357–64. doi:10.1097/PSY.0b013e3181d9523c.

Metabolic Syndrome

"About Metabolic Syndrome." American Heart Association, August 16, 2012. http://www.heart.org/HEARTORG/Conditions/More/MetabolicSyndrome /About-Metabolic-Syndrome_UCM_301920_Article.jsp.

Alberti, K. G. M. M., P. Zimmet, and J. Shaw. "Metabolic Syndrome–a New World-wide Definition. A Consensus Statement from the International Diabetes Federation." *Diabetic Medicine* 23, no. 5 (2006): 469–80. doi:10.1111/j.1464-5491.2006.01858.x.

Hu, G., Q. Qiao, J. Tuomilehto, et al. "Plasma Insulin and Cardiovascular Mortality in Non-Diabetic European Men and Women: A Meta-Analysis of Data from Eleven Prospective Studies." *Diabetologia* 47, no. 7 (2004). doi:10.1007/s00125-004-1433-4.

Knowler, W. C., E. Barrett-Connor, S. E. Fowler, et al. "Reduction in the Incidence of Type 2 Diabetes with Lifestyle Intervention or Metformin." *New England Journal of Medicine* 346, no. 6 (February 07, 2002): 393–403. doi:10.1056/NEJMoa012512.

Pouliot, M. "Waist Circumference and Abdominal Sagittal Diameter: Best Simple Anthropometric Indexes of Abdominal Visceral Adipose Tissue Accumulation and Related Cardiovascular Risk in Men and Women." *American Journal of Cardiology* 73, no. 7 (March 1994): 460–8. doi:10.1016/ 0002-9149(94)90676-9.

Robins, S. J., H. B. Rubins, F. H. Faas, et al. "Insulin Resistance and Cardiovascular Events with Low HDL Cholesterol: The Veterans Affairs HDL Intervention Trial (VA-HIT)." *Diabetes Care* 26, no. 5 (2003): 1513–517. doi:10.2337/diacare.26.5.1513.

"Symptoms and Diagnosis of Metabolic Syndrome." American Heart Association, August 24, 2011. http://www.heart.org/HEARTORG/Conditions/More/MetabolicSyndrome/Symptoms-and -Diagnosis-of-Metabolic-Syndrome_UCM_301925_Article.jsp.

Vuguin, P. M., K. Hartil, M. Kruse, et al. "Shared Effects of Genetic and Intrauterine and Perinatal Environment on the Development of Metabolic Syndrome." *PLoS One* 8, no. 5 (May 2013).

"Why Metabolic Syndrome Matters." American Heart Association, March 29, 2012. http://www.heart.org/HEARTORG/Conditions/More/MetabolicSyndrome/ Why-Metabolic-Syndrome-Matters_UCM_301922_Article.jsp.

Thyroid Hormone Imbalance

Dugdale III, David. "Hypothyroidism." National Institutes of Health, June 4, 2012. http://www.nlm.nih.gov/medlineplus/ency/article/000353.htm.

Fox, C. S., M. J. Pencina, R. B. D'Agostino, et al. "Relations of Thyroid Function to Body Weight: Cross-Sectional and Longitudinal Observations in a Community-Based Sample." *Archives of Internal Medicine* 168, no. 6 (March 24, 2008): 587–92. doi:10.1001/archinte.168.6.587.

"Hyperthyroidism (Overactive Thyroid)." Mayo Clinic, November 20, 2012. http://www.mayoclinic.com/health/hyperthyroidism/DS00344.

"Hypothyroidism (Underactive Thyroid)." Mayo Clinic, December 1, 2012. http://www.mayoclinic.com/health/hypothyroidism/DS00353.

Estrogen Imbalance

American Chemical Society. "Revealing Estrogen's Secret Role in Obesity." News release, August 20, 2007. https://portal.acs.org/portal/acs/corg/memberapp?_nfpb=true&_pageLabel =PP_ARTICLEMAIN&node_id=222&content_id=CTP_006349&use_sec=true&sec_url_var =region1.

Davis, S. R., C. Castelo-Branco, P. Chedraui, et al. "Understanding Weight Gain at Menopause." *Climacteric* 15, no. 5 (October 2012): 419–29.

"Polycystic Ovary Syndrome (PCOS) Face Sheet." Womenshealth.gov, March 17, 2010. http://www .womenshealth.gov/publications/our-publications/fact-sheet/polycystic-ovary-syndrome.cfm#j.

"What is Perimenopause, Menopause, & Postmenopause?" Cleveland Clinic, May 2013, accessed June 20, 2013. http://my.clevelandclinic.org/disorders/menopause/hic-what-is-perimenopause -menopause-postmenopause.aspx.

Xu, Y., T. P. Nedungadi, L. Zhu, et al. "Distinct Hypothalamic Neurons Mediate Estrogenic Effects on Energy Homeostasis and Reproduction." *Cell Metabolism* 14, no. 4 (October 5, 2011): 453–65.

Sleep Disorders

Broussard, J. L., D. A. Ehrmann, E. Van Cauter, E. Tasali, and M. J. Brady. "Impaired Insulin Signaling in Human Adipocytes after Experimental Sleep Restriction: A Randomized, Crossover Study." *Annals of Internal Medicine* 157, no. 8 (October 16, 2012): 549–57.doi:10.7326/0003-4819-157 -8-201210160-00005.

Hogenkamp, P. S., E. Nilsson, V. C. NIlsson, et al. "Acute Sleep Deprivation Increases Portion Size and Affects Food Choice in Young Men."*Psychoneuroendocrinology* S0306-4530, no. 13 (February 18, 2013). doi:10.1016/j.psyneuen.2013.01.012.

"Insulin Resistance and Prediabetes." National Institute of Diabetes and Digestive and Kidney Diseases, NIH Pub no. 13-4893 (November 2012). http://diabetes.niddk.nih.gov/dm/pubs/insulinresistance/.

Klok, M. D., S. Jakobsdottir, and M. L. Drent. "The Role of Leptin and Ghrelin in the Regulation of Food Intake and Body Weight in Humans: A Review." *Obesity Reviews* 8, no. 1 (January 2007): 21–34.

Markwald, R. R., E. L. Melanson, M. R. Smith, et al. "Impact of Insufficient Sleep on Total Daily Energy Expenditure, Food Intake, and Weight Gain." *Proceedings of the National Academy of Sciences of the United States of America* 110, no. 14 (April 2013): 5695–700. doi:10.1073/pnas.1216951110.

"Obesity and Sleep." National Sleep Foundation, accessed May 16, 2013. http://www.sleepfoundation.org/article/sleep-topics/obesity-and-sleep.

Spiegel, K., E. Tasali, P. Penev, and E. Van Cauter. "Brief Communication: Sleep Curtailment in Healthy Young Men Is Associated with Decreased Leptin Levels, Elevated Ghrelin Levels, and Increased Hunger and Appetite." *Annals of Internal Medicine* 141, no. 11 (December 7, 2004): 846–50.

St-Onge, M. P., A. L. Roberts, J. Chen, et al. "Short Sleep Duration Increases Energy Intakes but Does Not Change Energy Expenditure in Normal-Weight Individuals." *American Journal of Clinical Nutrition* 94, no. 2 (August 2011): 410–6. doi:10.3945/ajcn.111.013904.

Yu, Winnie. "Eating Tips for Better Sleep." Cleveland Clinic Wellness Institute, September 8, 2009, accessed May 09, 2013. http://www.cleveland-clinicwellness.com/mind/BetterSleep/Pages/EatWellforSoundSleep.aspx.

Stress Fat/Cortisol Overproduction

Creagan, Edward T. "Stress and Weight Gain." Mayo Clinic, July 23, 2011. http://www.mayoclinic.com/health/stress/AN01128.

"How Stress Affects Your Health." American Psychological Association, 2013. http://www.apa.org/helpcenter/stress.aspx.

"Stress Affects Both Body and Mind." National Institutes of Health, January 2007. http://newsinhealth.nih.gov/2007/January/docs/01features_01.htm.

"Stress: Constant Stress Puts Your Health at Risk." Mayo Clinic, September 11, 2010. http://www.mayoclinic.com/health/stress/SR00001.

Digestive Tract Imbalance

"Gastroesophageal Reflux Disease." National Institutes of Health, August 2011. http://www.nlm.nih.gov/medlineplus/ency/article/000265.htm.

"Gastrointestinal Disorders." Cleveland Clinic, September 2008. http://my.clevelandclinic.org/disorders/gastrointestinal_tract_disorders/hic_gastrointestinal_disorders.aspx.

"GERD or Acid Reflux or Heartburn Overview." Cleveland Clinic. http://my.clevelandclinic.org/disorders/acid_reflux/dd_overview.aspx.

Gill, H., and J. Prasad. "Probiotics, Immunomodulation, and Health Benefits." *Advances in Experimental Medicine and Biology* 606 (2008): 423–54.

"What's the Difference between a Food Intolerance and Food Allergy?" Mayo Clinic, June 3, 2011. http://www.mayoclinic.com/health/food-allergy/AN01109.

Zeratsky, Katherine. "Is It Important to Include Probiotics and Prebiotics in a Healthy Diet?" Mayo Clinic, September 15, 2011. http://www.mayoclinic.com/health/probiotics/AN00389.

PART 5: Protecting Your Weight Loss for a Lifetime

Chapter 12   Maintaining Your Success: The Management Phase

"Americans Consume Too Much Sodium (Salt)." Centers for Disease Control and Prevention, February 24, 2011. http://www.cdc.gov/features/dssodium.

"Dietary Sodium." National Heart, Lung, and Blood Institute, May 2013. http://www.nlm.nih.gov /medlineplus/dietarysodium.html.

Mattes, R. D., and D. Donnelly. "Relative Contributions of Dietary Sodium Sources." *Journal of the American College of Nutrition* 10, no. 4 (August 1999): 383–93.

"Shaking the Salt Habit." American Heart Association, April 22, 2013. http://www.heart.org /HEARTORG/Conditions/HighBloodPressure/PreventionTreatmentofHighBloodPressure /Shaking-the-Salt-Habit_UCM_303241_Article.jsp.

Zeratsky, Katherine, RD, LD. "What's the Difference between Sea Salt and Table Salt?" Mayo Clinic, January 3, 2013. http://www.mayoclinic.com/health/sea-salt/AN01142.

Zieve, D. "Sodium in Diet." National Institutes of Health, June, 2012. http://www.nlm.nih.gov /medlineplus/ency/article/002415.htm.

Chapter 13   Your Return to Health

"A Heart-Healthy Diet Is Good for the Brain and Memory." American Heart Association, July 2, 2012, accessed May 09, 2013. http://www.heart.org/HEARTORG/Conditions/More /MyHeartand-StrokeNews/A-Heart-Healthy-Diet-is-Good-for-the-Brain-and-Memory _UCM_441866_Article.jsp.

"Adopt a Brain-Healthy Diet." Alzheimer's Association, accessed May 09, 2013. http://www.alz.org/we_can_help_adopt_a_brain_healthy_diet.asp.

"Aging Hearts and Arteries: A Scientific Quest." National Institute On Aging, April 2005. http://www.nia.nih.gov/health/publication/aging-hearts-and-arteries.

"Belly Fat in Women: Taking—and Keeping—It Off." Mayo Clinic, June 8, 2013. http://www.mayoclinic.com/health/belly-fat/WO00128.

Cecil, J. E., R. Tavendale, P. Watt, M. M. Hetherington, and C. N. Palmer. "An Obesity-Associated FTO Gene Variant and Increased Energy Intake in Children." *New England Journal of Medicine* 359, no. 24 (December 11, 2008): 2558–66. doi:10.1056/NEJMoa0803839.

Chen, Y., D. Rennie, Y. F. Cormier, and J. Dosman. "Waist Circumference Is Associated with Pulmonary Function in Normal-Weight, Overweight, and Obese Subjects." *American Journal of Clinical Nutrition* 85, no. 1 (January 2007): 35–9.

Church, C., L. Moir, F. McMurray, et al. "Overexpression of FTO Leads to Increased Food Intake and Results in Obesity." *Nature Genetics* 42, no. 12 (December 2010): 1086–92.

Ciolac, Emmanuel G. "High-Intensity Interval Training and Hypertension: Maximizing the Benefits of Exercise?" *American Journal of Cardiovascular Disease* 2, no. 2 (2012): 102–10.

Davis, S. R., C. Castelo-Branco, P. Chedraui, et al. "Understanding Weight Gain and Menopause." *Climacteric* 15, no. 5 (October 2012): 419–29. doi:10.3109./13697137.2012.707385.

"Dietary Fats: Know Which Types to Choose." Mayo Clinic, February 15, 2011. http://www.mayoclinic.com/health/fat/NU00262.

Do, R., C. Xie, X. Zhang, et al. "The Effect of Chromosome Variants on Cardiovascular Disease May Be Modified by Dietary Intake: Evidence from a Case/Control and Prospective Study." *PLoS Medicine* 8, no. 10 (October 2011): e1001106.

Donges, Cheyne E., Rob Duffield, and Eric J. Drinkwater. "Effects of Resistance or Aerobic Exercise Training on Interleukin-6, C-Reactive Protein, and Body Composition." *Medicine & Science in Sports & Exercise* 42, no. 2 (February 2010): 304–13. doi:10.1249/MSS.0b013e3181b117ca.

"Eating for Target Blood Glucose Levels (Your Guide to Diet and Diabetes)." University of Illinois Extension, accessed June 13, 2013. http://urbanext.illinois.edu/diabetes2/section.cfm?SectionID=3.

"Exercise: 7 Benefits of Regular Physical Activity." Mayo Clinic, July 23, 2011. http://www.mayoclinic.com/health/exercise/HQ01676.

Faria, A. N., F. F. Ribeiro Filho, S. R. Gouveia Ferreira, and M. T. Zanella. "Impact of Visceral Fat on Blood Pressure and Insulin Sensitivity in Hypertensive Obese Women." *Obesity Research* 10, no. 12 (December 2002): 1203–6.

Foster, G. D., H. R. Wyatt, J. O. Hill, et al. "Weight and Metabolic Outcomes after 2 Years on a Low-Carbohydrate versus Low-Fat Diet: A Randomized Trial." *Annals of Internal Medicine* 153, no. 3 (August 2010): 147–57.

Grandner, M. A., N. Jackson, J. R. Gerstner, and K. L. Knutson. "Dietary Nutrients Associated with Short and Long Sleep Duration. Data from a Nationally Representative Sample." *Appetite* 64 (May 2013): 71–80.

Gremeaux, V., J. Drigny, A. Nigam, et al. "Long-Term Lifestyle Intervention with Optimized High-Intensity Interval Training Improves Body Composition, Cardiometabolic Risk, and Exercise Parameters in Patients with Abdominal Obesity." *American Journal of Physical Medicine & Rehabilitation* 91, no. 11 (November 2012): 941–50.

Gómez-Pinilla, Fernando. "Brain Foods: The Effects of Nutrients on Brain Function." *Nature Reviews Neuroscience* 9, no. 7 (2008): 568–78. doi:10.1038/nrn2421.

"HDL Cholesterol: How to Boost Your 'Good' Cholesterol." Mayo Clinic, November 09, 2012, accessed May 09, 2013. http://www.mayoclinic.com/health/hdl-cholesterol/CL00030.

"Health Briefs: Alzheimer's Rate of Decline; Exercise and the 'Obesity Gene.'" Press of Atlantic City, January 28, 2012, accessed June 17, 2013. http://www.pressofatlanticcity.com/life/health-briefs-alzheimer-s-rate-of-decline-exercise -and-the/article_d081ba57-1a96-55d3-a7f4-adaf555e4837.html.

Herber-Gast, G. C., and G. D. Mishra. "Fruit, Mediterranean-Style, and High-Fat and -Sugar Diets are Associated with the Risk of Night Sweats and Hot Flashes in Midlife: Results from a Prospective Cohort Study." *American Journal of Clinical Nutrition* 97, no. 5 (May 2013): 1092–9.

Ho, A. J., J. L. Stein, X. Hua, et al. "From the Cover: A Commonly Carried Allele of the Obesity-Related FTO Gene Is Associated with Reduced Brain Volume in the Healthy Elderly." *Proceedings of the National Academy of Sciences* 107, no. 18 (April 19, 2010): 8404–09. doi:10.1073/pnas.0910878107.

"How Does Fiber Affect Blood Glucose Levels?" Joslin Diabetes Center, June 21, 2013. http://www.joslin.org/info/how_does_fiber_affect_blood_glucose_levels.html.

Imayama, I., C. M. Ulrich, S. M. Alfano, et al. "Effects of a Caloric Restriction Weight Loss Diet and Exercise on Inflammatory Biomarkers in Overweight/obese Postmenopausal Women: A Randomized Controlled Trial." *Cancer Research* 72, no. 9 (May 1, 2012): 2314–26. doi:10.1158/0008-5472.

Jenkins, D. J. A., P. J. H. Jones, B. Lamarche, et al. "Effect of a Dietary Portfolio of Cholesterol-Lowering Foods Given at 2 Levels of Intensity of Dietary Advice on Serum Lipids in Hyperlipidemia: A Randomized Controlled Trial." *JAMA: Journal of the American Medical Association* 306, no. 8 (2011): 831–9. doi:10.1001/jama.2011.1202.

Johns Hopkins Medicine. "Losing Weight, Especially in the Belly, Improves Sleep Quality, According to a Johns Hopkins Study." News release, November 6, 2012. http://www.hopkinsmedicine.org/news/media/releases/losing_weight_especially_in_the_belly_improves_sleep_quality_according_to_a_johns_hopkins_study.

Kanoski, Scott E., and Terry L. Davidson. "Western Diet Consumption and Cognitive Impairment: Links to Hippocampal Dysfunction and Obesity." *Physiology & Behavior* 103, no. 1 (2011): 59–68. doi:10.1016/j.physbeh.2010.12.003.

Kilpelainen, T. O., L. Qi, S. Brage, et al. "Physical Activity Attenuates the Influence of FTO variants on Obesity Risk: A Meta-Analysis of 218,166 adults and 19,268 Children." *PLoS Medicine* 8, no. 11 (November 2011): e1001116.

Klem, M. L., R. R. Wing, M. T. McGuire, H. M. Seagle, and J. O. Hill. "A Descriptive Study of Individuals Successful at Long-Term Maintenance of Substantial Weight Loss." *American Journal of Clinical Nutrition* 66, no. 2 (August 1997): 239–46.

Leone, N., D. Courbon, F. Thomas, et al. "Lung Function Impairment and Metabolic Syndrome: The Critical Role of Abdominal Obesity." *American Journal of Respiratory and Critical Care Medicine* 179, no. 6 (March 15, 2009): 509–16.

Little, J. P., J. B. Gillen, M. E. Percival, et al. "Low-Volume High-Intensity Interval Training Reduces Hyperglycemia and Increases Muscle Mitochondrial Capacity in Patients with Type 2 Diabetes." *Journal of Applied Physiology* 111, no. 6 (December 2011): 1554–60.

"Menopause: Staying Healthy through Good Nutrition." Cleveland Clinic. http://my.clevelandclinic.org/disorders/Menopause/hic_Menopause_Staying_Healthy_Through_Good_Nutrition.aspx.

"Menopause Weight Gain: Stop the Middle Age Spread." Mayo Clinic, June 11, 2013, accessed June 13, 2013. http://www.mayoclinic.com/health/menopause-weight-gain/HQ01076/NSECTIONGROUP=2.

North, C. J., C. S. Venter, and J. C. Jerling. "The Effects of Dietary Fibre on C-reactive Protein, an Inflammation Marker Predicting Cardiovascular Disease." *European Journal of Clinical Nutrition* 63, no. 8 (2009): 921–33. doi:10.1038/ejcn.2009.8.

Ohlson, Melissa. "7 Helpful Tips for Sustaining Energy Throughout the Day." Cleveland Clinic. http://my.clevelandclinic.org/be_well/fatigue_fighting_foods_bewell209.aspx.

Rankin, J. W., and A. D. Turpyn. "Low Carbohydrate, High Fat Diet Increases C-Reactive Protein during Weight Loss." *Journal of the American College of Nutrition* 26, no. 2 (April 2007): 163–9.

Reid, K. J., K. G. Baron, B. Lu, et al. "Aerobic Exercise Improves Self-Reported Sleep and Quality of Life in Older Adults with Insomnia." *Sleep Medicine* 11, no. 9 (October 2010): 934–40. doi:10.1016/j.sleep.2010.04.014.

Riccardi, G., and A. A. Rivellese. "Effects of Dietary Fiber and Carbohydrate on Glucose and Lipoprotein Metabolism in Diabetic Patients." *Diabetes Care* 14, no. 12 (1991): 1115–25. doi:10.2337/diacare.14.12.1115.

Riserus, U., W. Willett, and F. Hu. "Dietary Fats and Prevention of Type 2 Diabetes." *Progress in Lipid Research* 48, no. 1 (2009): 44–51. doi:10.1016/j.plipres.2008.10.002.

Salome, C. M., G. G. King, and N. Berend. "Physiology of Obesity and Effects on Lung Function." *Journal of Applied Physiology* 108, no. 1 (January 2010): 206–11. doi:10.1152/japplphysiol.00694 .2009.

Schwartz, Jay. "The Normal Values for Post Exercise Heart Rates." AZcentral, accessed June 13, 2013. http://healthyliving.azcentral.com/normal-values-post-exercise-heart-rates-7220.html.

Sharma, S., M. F. Fernandes, and S. Fulton. "Adaptations in Brain Reward Circuitry Underlie Palatable Food Cravings and Anxiety Induced by High-Fat Diet Withdrawal." *International Journal of Obesity*, December 11, 2012. doi:10.1038/ijo.2012.197.

Sulzer, Jesse. "How Does BMI Affect the Heart Rate Response to Exercise?" AZcentral. http://healthyliving.azcentral.com/bmi-affect-heart-rate-response-exercise-1295.html.

Suzuki, S., M. Kojima, S. Tokudome, et al. "Obesity/Weight Gain and Breast Cancer Risk: Findings from the Japan Collaborative Cohort Study for the Evaluation of Cancer Risk." *Journal of Epidemiology* 23, no. 2 (2013): 139–45.

"10 Ways to Control High Blood Pressure without Medication." Mayo Clinic, July 19, 2012, accessed May 09, 2013. http://www.mayoclinic.com/health/high-blood-pressure/HI00027.

Trapp, E. G., D. J. Chisholm, J. Freund, and S. H. Boutcher. "The Effects of High-Intensity Intermittent Exercise Training on Fat Loss and Fasting Insulin Levels of Young Women." *International Journal of Obesity* 32, no. 4 (2008): 684–91. doi:10.1038/sj.ijo.0803781.

Villaverde-Gutierrez, C., E. Araujo, F. Cruz, et al. "Quality of Life of Rural Menopausal Women in Response to Customized Exercise Programme." *Journal of Advanced Nursing* 54, no. 1 (April 2006): 11–19.

Vimaleswaran, K. S., S. Li, J. H. Zhao, et al. "Physical Activity Accentuates the Body Mass Index-Increasing Influence of Genetic Variation in the FTO Gene." *American Journal of Clinical Nutrition* 90, no. 2. (August 2009): 425–8.

"Ways to Boost Your HDL Cholesterol." Johns Hopkins Health Alerts, April 24, 2009, accessed May 09, 2013. http://www.johnshopkinshealthalerts.com/reports/heart_health/3028-1.html.

Yasmeen, Rumana. "Role of Vitamin a Metabolism in Visceral Obesity." PhD diss., Ohio State University, 2012.

"Your Guide to Lowering Your Blood Pressure with DASH." US Department of Health and Human Services, April 2006. http://www.nhlbi.nih.gov/health/public/heart/hbp/dash/new_dash.pdf.

Yu, Winnie. "Eating Tips for Better Sleep." Cleveland Clinic Wellness Institute, September 8, 2009, accessed May 09, 2013. http://www.cleveland-clinicwellness.com/mind/BetterSleep/Pages/EatWellforSoundSleep.aspx.